Intermitte

Eat what you love, heal your body, and improve your health through this secret weight loss guide! Living an healthy lifestyle, burn fat, and losing pounds at the same time has never been so simple! (Beginners friendly)

By Serena Baker

Table of Contents

Foreword

For anyone seeking a boost into health or a bit of assistance losing some pesky weight—for anyone hoping to find renewed energy or better weight maintenance—for anyone struggling with food, strength, nutrition, or overall health, this book is made just for you.

Intermittent Fasting: Eat what you love, heal your body, and improve your health through this secret weight loss guide! Living an healthy lifestyle, burn fat, and losing pounds at the same time has never been so simple! Is a project I've been working on for a while, and I congratulate you for downloading it now as it has reached its perfection and completion. In this book, I aim to bring my education, experiences, and passions together to help readers reach all their fitness, dietary, and healthy goals.

My name is Serena Baker, and I graduated a few years ago with a bachelor's degree in Nutrition. I have been working since then to compile health and fitness books for anyone devoted on the path to personal growth. In this book specifically, my passion for fitness focuses on healthy diet and lifestyle first and foremost. I practice Intermittent Fasting in my own life and see consistent results regarding overall health, weight maintenance, and hunger level. So, I'm eager to share some tips of the trade with you. I'm excited to help as many people as I possibly can.

The chapters in this book will touch on everything about Intermittent Fasting, from the history of IF to the science behind it. The hard and fast facts, helpful recipes, ways to troubleshoot any issues, the different methods to try, ways to avoid hardship, and so much more. By the end of this book, you should find that you're confident about what IF is as well as what it will do for you once you start practicing it in your life, and you should have a plan set out to be able to do just that.

While many different books with this focus are available for a download, you've chosen this one, and I am both grateful and excited for you. Thank you for choosing this one, and I hope you look forward to all the good changes that are sure to be coming your way once you embrace Intermittent Fasting for yourself. Congratulations again, and good luck!

Introduction: The History of Intermittent Fasting

Within the past few years, the concept of Intermittent Fasting has started to trend heavily, impacting anyone interested in dieting and healthy living. Its origins, however, are much more ancient than most of us would ever think. In this chapter, you'll be introduced to the long history of Intermittent Fasting so that you can better understand how that trajectory leads to today. By the end of this section, you should feel confident that you know where the tradition came from, as well as what it has to do with you—reading this book in this very moment.

IF for Primitive Humans

Intermittent Fasting has been a practice as long as humans have existed. In the times of our most primitive ancestors, IF wasn't so much a chosen lifestyle as it was a necessity. It came down to the prevalence and availability of food—and the hunter's and gatherer's abilities to acquire it.

In these ancient times, people would have had to go longer between meals and sometimes perhaps spend days without eating. However, what arose from necessity produced incredible and even sustainable physical, mental, and emotional effects. These ancient people would have also (likely unintentionally) been able to concentrate better, live longer, slowing age and digest with ease consistently.

Primitive humans would also occasionally fast for shared purposes once societies and civilizations started assembling. For instance, before going off to war, communities would fast, and young people coming-of-age would fast as part of those rituals. Sometimes societies would also demand a fast as an offering to the gods or to implore the end of natural disasters such as floods or famines.

Religious Instances of IF

On the same vein as using a fast as an offering to the gods, many ancient cultures eventually required some fasting for their religion purposes. Consider Christianity. Orthodox Christians of the Greek variety still practice their ancient fasts, which comprise almost 200 days out of the year. Non-Orthodox Christians are also invited to fast whenever moved to do so to become closer to the Holy Trinity.

Consider Buddhism. The practice of intermittent fasting has always been essential to reaching enlightenment, because it helps the soul undo its ropes to the body. The enlightened one, Siddhartha, practiced fasting for many years as a method to acquire wisdom.

Consider Judaism. The day before Passover, it is an ancient tradition followed still today that the first-born child of each family should fast to celebrate the miracle from Moses' time that spared all Hebrew first-borns. Furthermore, Jewish people are invited to fast throughout the year at any point to celebrate a life lost, to appeal to God or a prophet, or to express sorrow for a sin or wrong committed.

Consider Islam. The holy month of Ramadan features a 4-week-long fast from the time the sun rises to the time the sun sets. During this time, drinks are also shunned, as well as alcohol drinking, smoking, or performing any bad habits or repetitive practices that don't serve the soul. Muhammad, the prophet of Islam, also suggested his followers fast every Monday and Thursday (essentially the 5:2 method, which we'll address in chapter 6!), but it's unclear how consistently this suggestion is heeded.

Other religions across the world have also required a temporary fast for spiritual reasons, and it is true that many have gotten closer to their gods through this practice. However, there are so many more benefits to fasting than just these spiritual ones, and these other applications are made clear in the next chapters.

From the Past to Now

On top of being used for survival and religious purposes, intermittent fasting has gained appeal through time for its medical applications as well. Even millennia before its trending popularity today, back in 400 BC, intermittent fasting made an appearance and gained popularity by the suggestion of Hippocrates.

Yes, *that* Hippocrates! The infamous "father of modern medicine" advocated for fasting to heal almost any internal injury or state of disease. He once wrote, "To eat when you are sick, is to feed your illness," if that gives you any indication of the incredible uses he found for the practice.

Other ancient Greek philosophers, writers, and historians have echoed these concepts from Hippocrates through time into the early years, AD. Essentially, just like how animals seem to "fast" when they're getting sick or feeling unwell, humans have the same instincts but often ignore them, pushing through the illness and feeding it with food when the body needs the exact opposite.

Past the ancient Greeks, however, other thinkers across time have affirmed the same feelings. For example, Paracelsus (another founder of modern medicine) famously wrote, "Fasting is the greatest remedy," and Benjamin Franklin (one of America's founding fathers) also once inscribed in a journal, "The best of all medicines is resting and fasting."

In the past, fasting has also been used as a form of political protest, and the most famous instance of this happening occurred with Mahatma Gandhi, who lasted 21 days at his longest period of fasting. His goals were to protest against India's dependence on Britain and to acquire freedom and integrity for his people. Many others have taken up fasting for similar aims, but none have been so successful or so famous, it seems.

Contemporary Applications

Now, it seems that fasting has gained new fame in the form of Intermittent Fasting, and the capital letters here are used intentionally to connote the almost "patented" application of these ancient theories in relation to health and weight loss in recent times.

This practice of Intermittent Fasting has been trending for the past few years, and its impact has spread widely since then. People have lost incredible amounts of weight. They've seen their energy levels improve drastically. They've been able to heal brain disorders and reverse the signs of aging. People across the world have come to understand what amazing uses fasting can have, and they are becoming healthier because of these realizations.

Doctors who have practiced fasting cures for decades have almost consistently welcomed the increased interest in IF these days, for they know how much good this practice can do for so many. Fasting is still used for religious and spiritual purposes, and some still practice it as they strive to survive. For others, IF today is revered as the so-called "fountain of youth," and many dietary plans are starting to incorporate its themes.

Overall, it seems that IF has been used throughout time for three main things: survival, spiritual connection, and body/mind health. These applications are valid today, but the focus tends toward that final point in the list: body/mind health. For those seeking a state of internal balance, IF can be a blessing. For those intrigued by IF, keep reading to find out more and to learn how to build this practice into your daily routine.

Chapter 1: Explaining Intermittent Fasting

What is Intermittent Fasting about after all, and how the heck does it work? This chapter will answer these questions and more. By the end of it, you should have a solid grasp on the practice of Intermittent Fasting, and you should also have a sense of why it's trending so much these days (as well as whether or not it sounds right for you).

What it Is

Intermittent Fasting is essentially the practice of restricting mealtimes, reducing snacking, or cutting out days of eating, based on the method one chooses. One of the most popular IF methods is 5:2, which is to eat five days a week and fast the other two. Others focus on eating windows and fasting periods within each day. The easiest method to start with for IF, however, is just to stop eating snacks.

So many of us snack unconsciously or when we're getting moody without any real hunger. So many of us eat unconsciously in general, and then we're confused why our bodies are holding onto the weight. Intermittent Fasting reminds the body what food is for, and it restarts that nutritional absorption potential. All you have to do is cut out the snacks, fast a few hours a day, or just drink water a few days a week.

IF is both a dietary choice and a lifestyle, but those who have the most success with IF will tell you that it became a lifestyle for them almost instantly. Sure, dieting plans and IF can match up nicely, but for some, IF requires no dietary change whatsoever.

The point is to eat less and to eat less often. The brain and the body will respond in no time.

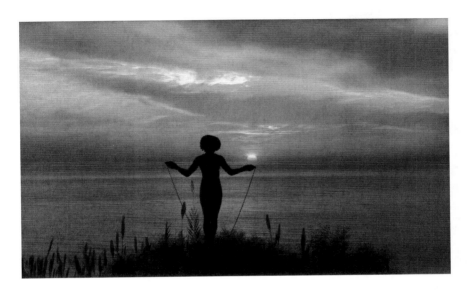

How it Works

There is a lot of science behind why IF works, and that will be detailed in chapter 4, but for now, it will suffice to say that IF works because it restricts the body of toxins and allows itself to clear out any excess. It gives the body a break and provides a moment to recalibrate, basically. And with this recalibration, neurotransmitters are released easier in the brain, and one's senses of hungry and full are adjusted back to how they should be. Once the food is eaten after the fast, too, nutritional absorption is boosted throughout the entire body, to the benefit of all one's organs.

Additionally, Intermittent Fasting recalibrates one's hormones in relation to stress and hunger so that balanced mood, patience, and intellect can be increased despite the seeming lack of food.

IF tells the brain and body to restart. It makes your system go back to basics and clean out any gunk, and a lot of that gunk tends to be stored fat or water weight. It sees the toxins in your body and refuses to let you hold onto them. Overall, IF proves that a change in routine can have great and lasting effects on one's health.

Why People Start

People most often start Intermittent Fasting because they're interested in losing that pesky and lingering weight. They're trying to lose the holiday pounds, or they're interested in slimming down for beach season. Others are trying to let go of tens, if not hundreds, of pounds through this lifestyle shift. Basically, people most often start due to weight.

On the other hand, people have been known to start IF for the sake of reversing aging, healing the heart, or healing the brain. These effects will be detailed further in chapter 11! But for now, simply know that IF can restart a lot of systems in the body, not just the digestive and endocrine systems. IF can affect the hormones that contribute to aging, the ease with which blood flows through one's veins and arteries, and the potential for the brain to heal itself with increased plasticity.

As one final point, some people start IF because they're not satisfied with the bodies they're working to sculpt at the gym. Sometimes, people aren't particularly heavy, they're just hefty, and they're working on slimming down in the right places and bulking up in others. For these people, IF can help to repurpose lingering fat to either be burned for energy, or turned to muscle.

Why People Stay

People *start* Intermittent Fasting for a variety of reasons, but they always *stay* for the same reason, which is that the effects are undeniable and incredible. Regardless of why you start, you will stay because you will see changes in your body that you like, appreciate, and value. You will stay because you will have proven yourself strong in many ways and you will undoubtedly like what you've learned about yourself.

You will stay because IF will have helped you grow in ways you never imagined. Whether your goals were weight loss, anti-aging effects, sharper cognition, better memory, less disease, or otherwise, you will surely see that Intermittent Fasting can turn things around. All you need to do is devote some determination, a pinch of commitment, and a good lot of will power to the cause. Then, the sky's the limit, and your health is well within reach.

Chapter 2: Getting to the Facts

Before you know whether or not Intermittent Fasting will be right for you, it helps to go through the common myths, mistakes, and side-effects associated with this dietary choice and lifestyle. This chapter will do exactly that for you, and by the end, you should have most (if not all) of your concerns addressed.

8 Myths about IF Busted

There's a lot of misinformation circulating about Intermittent Fasting, but the truth is out there, too! Here are 8 myths about Intermittent Fasting and their respective *realities*.

1. MYTH: <u>Your body will definitely enter in starvation mode</u>.

   BUSTED: Your body will *not* definitely enter in starvation mode through Intermittent Fasting. Skipping meals or adjusting to longer periods between meals where you don't eat is not going to make you starve. It's going to help your body remember how to absorb nutrients. It's going to help you thrive instead.

2. MYTH: <u>You'll lose muscle in this endeavor</u>.

   BUSTED: This myth goes along the same lines as the first one, above. Just like your body won't enter the starvation mode (unless something goes very, very wrong or you're trying to do too much); your body won't lose muscle through IF. The only reason why IF *would* cause muscle loss would be if it was causing you to starve, but once again, the first myth addresses this falsity, making this myth false as well.

3. MYTH: <u>You'll almost assuredly overeat during eating windows, and that's not healthy at all</u>.

BUSTED: While some people will have the *instinct* to overeat during eating windows, not everyone will overeat. Even those who do at the start will realize how to move forward without this overeating instinct in the future. Your body will urge you to overeat because, at the start, it won't realize what you're doing to it, but as long as you keep portion sizes largely the same and don't gorge on snacks, your body will adjust and so will your appetite.

4. MYTH: <u>Your metabolism will slow down dangerously</u>.

BUSTED: This myth is also addressed in chapter 12's Questions & Answers, but the point is that your metabolism won't slow down just because you're eating less often. People who think this myth is true, only assume that restricted caloric intake will make one's metabolism slow down over time, but these individuals forget that IF isn't *necessarily* about cutting down calories overall (although methods like 20:4 don't leave much room for full caloric intake). It's actually about cutting down the *times* during which one consumes calories. There needn't be any caloric restriction whatsoever! It just depends on the practitioner and what he or she decides to do with dieting in addition to IF.

5. MYTH: <u>You'll only *gain* weight if you try skipping meals</u>.

BUSTED: This myth is based on the same logic that drives myth #3 about overeating. If you gorge yourself during your eating windows, you'll surely gain weight, but hardly anyone will continuously gorge with IF. Anyone who tries will realize how unsuccessful it is, so he or she will not *continuously* gorge in response. Anyone who doesn't realize his or her efforts with eating are unsuccessful will soon realize that something's wrong, as his or her weight shows no improvement. Skipping meals never *necessarily* means that someone will gain weight. It just means that people who skip meals *and gorge or overeat* when it *is* mealtime won't see the desired effects.

6. MYTH: <u>During fast periods, you literally can't eat anything</u>.

   BUSTED: This myth is partially true and partially false. It's true only for methods like 12:12, 14:10, 16:8, and 20:4 that require fasting and eating in alternation within each individual day. For 12:12 method, for example, you'd spend 12 hours fasting and 12 hours eating. In this case, you would definitely not eat anything or consume any calories during that 12-hour fasting window, but the same isn't true for methods that alternate between days "on" and days "off" between fasting and eating. For those types of methods, you absolutely can eat during fasting periods! It might feel counterintuitive as you read these words, but you don't explicitly have to eat *nothing* during fast periods. Most methods that have full days of fasting actually allow for caloric intake as long as it's restricted by 20-25% of one's normal intake. Therefore, for methods like 5:2, alternate-day, eat-stop-eat, and crescendo, on days when you're fasting, you can still consume around 500 calories, and that will help a lot!

7. MYTH: <u>There's only one way to do IF that's right and truly the best.</u>

BUSTED: This myth is absolutely and utterly false. There is no one right way to practice Intermittent Fasting, and part of the beauty of IF is that there *are* so many different methods, meaning each approaching IF likely has a few different options to choose from. Similarly, different body and personality types will be drawn to different methods, based on individuals' abilities and goals. IF is about flexibility, adjustment, and self-correction. There's no one right method for everyone, and there's no "best" method to strive for. Do whatever method feels right and suits your life, and once you've found it, practice it as long as you can! That's far more realistic and accessible.

8. MYTH: <u>It's not natural to fast like that.</u>

BUSTED: It's more natural to practice Intermittent Fasting than it is to eat three full meals each day! It's more connected to our evolutionary drives and to our primitive selves to eat like this. And it's better for our brains, hearts, cells, and digestive systems to have a break from food once in a while to recalibrate. As you learned in the Introduction, people have been practicing Intermittent Fasting as long as humans have been in existence. It's only myths like this that circulate today that make it seem like IF is foreign, unhealthy, and dangerous. Animals of all types become healthier after periods of fasting, and humans are no different. Remember that we are animals and that IF is in our nature. Proceed with that confidence and knowledge!

4 Most Common Mistakes & How to Avoid Them

Given the number of people who have tried Intermittent Fasting, there's no reason why you should have to suffer through the most common mistakes! Here are 4 of the most common mistakes and how to properly avoid them.

1. Make sure you're breaking fast correctly! Many people make the mistake of breaking fast with something high in calories or with a really big serving or a portion of their favorite food. However, breaking fast should be a thoughtful and almost meditative event that's not about gorging, feeling full, or rushing to eat. Breaking fast, especially if it's been a long time since you've eaten, should be slow and respectful, to both the food and to your body. Don't cram in the calories or eat a lot right away! Your body doesn't want *or need* that type of treatment. Start with a small something or eat slowly through a big portion, so that your body can adjust without cramps or aches and pains. Be thoughtful and don't rush to avoid this common mistake.

2. Make sure you don't waste your eating window! Some people turn to Intermittent Fasting because their days are hectic already and it makes sense not to eat all the time. Sometimes, people choose small eating windows, particularly because they don't normally eat a lot each day, to begin with. For people who make these sorts of choices especially, please be careful to don't waste valuable eating time! It might seem like you can work forever and push off eating until later and later and later, but sometimes, you could push it off until the eating window is totally gone, and your body certainly won't

thank you for that. Be mindful of your timing and of when you're supposed to eat. Respect that allotment of time for what it can give to your body: health, nourishment, and energy.

3. <u>Make sure you don't try too much at once</u>! Some people try to fast while dieting while seriously exercising, and they wonder why they have no energy left! People who *want* to live high-intensity lifestyles like this are best suited toward plans like 5:2 (making sure not to exercise on those two fast days!). But even so, these individuals shouldn't put their bodies through *too much* stress with the addition of Intermittent Fasting. If you are attempting to do all three (diet, fast, and exercise), and you notice your energy level dropping, your mood swinging, or your belly burning, it might be time to cut back on one of those elements. Do a little less exercise! Eat a little more when you can! Try to add in some more calories! IF isn't about starvation, and it should never lead to that when done correctly and with healthy intentions. Remember that as you proceed with your journey.

4. <u>Make sure you don't give up too soon</u>! It's often the case that people give up on IF before the first week is over. They're frustrated by these feelings of hunger, and they feel convinced they'll never see results. Don't be duped into this way of thinking! Remember the power of your will. Be stubborn! Push through that first week and look forward to seeing results. They sometimes aren't as immediate as you'd hope, but that doesn't mean they're not coming! Even if you can tell the method you chose isn't working, try to last out the first week before troubleshooting and choosing a different one. For people

who aren't convinced even after switching methods, try to go a whole two weeks before giving up entirely. You never know—it could be that last day in two weeks that your body starts to show results! Keep a focused mindset and a clear eye on your goals. Push through any hardship and be stubborn with your hopes and actions! Success will come in time.

6 Unexpected Side-Effects of IF

Some of the side-effects of Intermittent Fasting are easily assumed, but some are far more unexpected. This section details six of the most commonly unexpected side-effects associated with the practice.

1. Irritability is one of the most commonly unexpected side-effects from Intermittent Fasting, but it is very prevalent, especially for people just beginning to transition into the lifestyle. People get angry! It's a thing. People get snippy and sassy when they're waiting for food. Unfortunately, this will be you, but you're definitely going to learn a lot about yourself during this period, and you'll eventually grow *through* these irritable feelings. Be patient with yourself (and especially patient with others). The irritability will fade, I promise.

2. Feeling cold is another of those things none of us would likely expect about from practicing Intermittent Fasting (or maybe it is, and I'm just off on this one!). You will probably feel extra sensitive to the cold through your fingers and toes while you're fasting, but this side-effect is totally normal! Don't be alarmed when you feel it. Instead, just know that it means your body is burning fat

and your blood sugar is decreasing, and these effects are standard and healthy to experience. Drink a little extra hot tea or wear a few extra layers to help keep warm.

3. Heartburn is a more uncommon side-effect of Intermittent Fasting, but it's another thing that's totally natural. Your stomach is used to producing acids to digest the foods you're consuming, and when you start adjusting to IF, these acids are being produced at times when you're potentially fasting, causing heartburn or reflux issues. With time, this side-effect should be mitigated if not totally alleviated. Keep drinking water and try not to eat foods that are super greasy or spicy when you do breakfast. If things don't get better, consider speaking with your doctor or nutritionist.

4. Bloating is a side-effect related to #5 below, Constipation. When you transition into Intermittent Fasting, your stomach is going to be processing things in a way that it hasn't in a long, long time—possibly ever. There will be weird side-effects like this for some, but it's all part of that adjustment period, and these issues should resolve themselves in a week or so. Drink a lot of water to aid the situation!

5. Constipation is related to Bloating, and it's just one of those things that might happen in your body as you get used to eating less or at incredibly different times than normal. Remember to drink a lot of water so whatever *is* in your system has enough hydration to come out without stress. Within a few weeks, the water cure (drink A LOT!!!) should help flush out the issue.

6. <u>More frequent urination</u> is common as well, and this situation most often arises due to the displacement of eating for the sake of the fast. During these fast periods, individuals are invited to drink anything (that doesn't have too many calories), and this often translates to a full bladder almost constantly—at least in the beginning! When things get tough, you'll want to drink more water. If things get gurgle-y or constipated on the inside, you'll want to drink more water. If you have headaches or get lightheaded, you'll want some water with a pinch of salt. If you need energy, you'll grab the coffee. You get the picture. Expect frequent bathroom runs.

Chapter 3: Benefits of Intermittent Fasting

There are so many incredible benefits possible for you once you choose Intermittent Fasting, and this chapter is dedicated to those individual benefits. First, we will go through 20 general positive points that arise from Intermittent Fasting, and then we will address five specific benefits each, for women and then for men, respectively. At the end of this section, you should feel excited by all the possibilities provided by IF, and you should be much better able to tell whether or not this lifestyle is right for you.

20 General Benefits

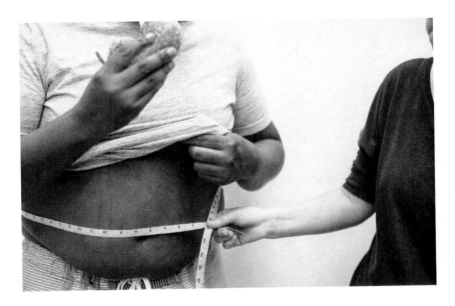

Intermittent Fasting has such incredible potential for so many different body and personality types, and 20 of the coolest benefits are listed below.

1. Incredible weight loss potential

2. Lowered insulin & blood sugar levels

3. Increased preservation of muscle mass

4. Increased neuroplasticity

5. Cancer healing potential

6. Lower blood pressure

7. Lower cholesterol

8. Overall longer life

9. Restructured nutrition absorption potential

10. Overall increased feeling of well-being

11. More energy for more tasks and activities

12. Improved cognition and mental processing

13. Better memory access and potential

14. Increased sense of welfare

15. High degree of independence and autonomy in choosing one's strategy or method

16. Overall ease in starting and maintaining one's approach

17. Increased (sense of) will power

18. Better ability to tune in with one's body

19. Increased awareness of the effects of food on the body, mind, and emotions

20. Ability to eat the same things and still lose weight

5 Benefits for Women in Specific

For women specifically, Intermittent Fasting poses certain trials and opportunities. Here are 5 of the most exciting benefits women can expect to see.

1. Lessened period cramps

2. Regulated or relieved process of menstruation

3. The potential for restricted fertility (this is a benefit for some!) at least during fast periods

4. Reduced internal inflammation that would lead to cancers of the reproductive organs

5. Better hormone regulation and healthier production

5 Benefits for Men in Specific

For men specifically, Intermittent Fasting can do a few different things than it can for women, and 5 of the best benefits are listed below.

1. Increased testosterone levels

2. Reduction of lingering estrogen levels from foods

3. Increases HGH (the Human Growth Hormone)

4. Reduced internal inflammation that would lead to prostate or renal cancer

5. Increased virility and sexual stamina overall

Chapter 4: The Science of Intermittent Fasting

You've learned a lot about Intermittent Fasting so far, but you still likely don't understand *why* it all works so well for dieting and health. This chapter is the antidote to that confusion! You will learn how Intermittent Fasting affect the body, how it interacts with diabetes, heart health, aging, and finally, the female body. By the end of this chapter, you should feel both highly informed about IF and aware of a few potential complications.

How IF Affects the Body

When you're feeling hungry, your body is under the sway of two very important hormones: leptin and ghrelin, and Intermittent Fasting affects both of those hormones substantially. In a typical situation, leptin decreases sensations of being hungry, and ghrelin makes you feel hungry instead. While leptin is secreted from fat cells throughout the body, ghrelin is only secreted from the stomach's lining. Together, leptin and ghrelin communicate with the brain's hypothalamus, telling the body when to stop or start eating. During IF, these hormones are released less often, causing the body to have a whole different experience of hunger and fullness.

Another important hormone in the context of eating and hunger suppression is insulin itself. The pancreas produces insulin, and it regulates how much glucose exists in our blood. Ultimately, high or low amounts of insulin affect the individual's weight greatly. Too little insulin and one can't keep weight on. Too much insulin and one can't lose weight whatsoever. While it seems that lower insulin is desired, there has to be a healthy balance, for *too low* insulin is actually disastrous for the body since glucose (or blood sugar) is a large part of how the body gets energy.

One final influencer of the body's hunger and weight loss situation is the individual's thyroid. If the thyroid is overactive, metabolism will work quickly, and energy, health, and weight will be affected. Conversely, an underactive thyroid will slow metabolism, energy, and health, and it will contribute to increased weight.

In the end, Intermittent Fasting affects the individual's weight by varying the production of these three important hormones and by working with the thyroid's natural potential. Essentially, those practicing IF will trigger these hormones to be released less often (or more consistently if the person is obese or diabetic to start with) due to the less-frequent eating schedule. Eventually, even the thyroid's effects should become balanced out through this altered eating schedule.

IF and Diabetes

For people with diabetes, Intermittent Fasting poses certain risks as well as incredible benefits. People with diabetes have altered insulin levels compared to the non-diabetic person, due to insulin resistance in their bodies. People with Type 1 diabetes cannot make insulin. They need to take insulin daily to have the energy and vigor to live. People with Type 2 diabetes have bodies that don't produce much insulin or don't use that insulin well at all.

With these altered productions of insulin, the blood sugar levels of the body have no way to be regulated, meaning that there's more standing glucose in the blood at all times with no way for it to get into the cells to be used for natural and physical energy. This higher blood sugar level can cause additional problems for the individual over time, but there is no legitimate cure other than taking insulin daily.

Intermittent Fasting, however, can provide a temporary cure when applied correctly in the lives of diabetic individuals (whose diabetic conditions are not severe). When IF is done on a daily basis with just a few fasting hours a day, people with diabetes show improved weight, blood sugar levels, and standing glucose levels. These individuals are not recommended to skip entire meals or fast for days at a time. Also, is not recommended for these people to strictly diet while they're applying IF. Instead, it works better to make food portions smaller and to eat fewer snacks in between.

IF and Heart Health

Heart health is a complicated issue in today's world. We all want to be healthy and thrive, but the foods we eat and the activities we engage in often don't align with those goals, and those more immediate actions win out. In effect, many of our hearts aren't as healthy as they could be. Heart disease is still the biggest killer in the world to this day. However, the introduction of Intermittent Fasting into someone's lifestyle can greatly alter this potential, for it can reduce many risks associated with heart disease.

For example, recent studies done on animals have proved that the practice of Intermittent Fasting improves numerous risk factors for heart disease. Some of these improvements include lowered cholesterol, reduced inflammation in the body, balanced blood sugar levels, and lower blood pressure. Essentially, IF won't cure heart disease, but it will reduce several risk factors that may exist in one's body (with or without him or her knowing).

When it comes down to it, as long as one's Intermittent Fasting experience involves the reintroduction of electrolytes into the body, there's no potential harm posed to the heart whatsoever. There's only potential for growth, bolstering, and strengthening. However, without the right reintroduction of electrolytes, there *is* still the possibility of heart palpitations in individuals attempting IF. The heart needs electrolytes for its stability and efficacy, so as long as you drink a bit of salt with your water, your heart will only thank you!

IF and Aging

People love to talk about how Intermittent Fasting can reverse the effects of aging, and they're not wrong! The tricky part is elucidating the science behind the process they're referencing. The anti-aging potential tied up with Intermittent Fasting applies mostly to two things: 1) your brain and 2) your whole body, through what's called "autophagy."

Overall, Intermittent Fasting heals the body through its ability to rejuvenate the cells. With this restricted caloric intake due to eating schedule or timing, the body's cells can function with less limitation and confusion while producing more energy for the body to use. In effect, the cells function more efficiently while the body can burn more fat and take in more oxygen for the organs and blood, encouraging the individual to live longer with increased sensations of "youth."

About those two original examples, Intermittent Fasting has been proven 1) to keep the brain fit and agile. It improves overall cognitive function and memory capacity as well as cleverness, wit, and quick, clear thinking in the moment. Furthermore, Intermittent Fasting 2) keeps the cells fit and agile through autophagy (which is kickstarted by IF), where the cells are encouraged to clean themselves up and get rid of any "trash" that might be clogging up the works. By just restricting your eating schedule a little bit each day (or each week), you can find your brain power boosted and your body ready for anything.

IF and the Female Body

Intermittent Fasting requires a different technique than most diets do, which is why it's more often referred to as a lifestyle. Additionally, this variance means that the effects of IF on the female body are a little different than the effects of the standard diet. For instance, dieting will easily cause weight loss in most people, but IF is a little trickier and much less consistent for women especially.

The female body, being created with birthing potential, has specific needs that are altered through an Intermittent Fasting eating schedule. With less hormones being released (which tell women when they are hungry and full) there is less fat being stored in their bodies and less fertility when it comes to their later aims of reproducing. In combination with a strict diet that counts calories or restricts fats, Intermittent Fasting can be dangerous for women of all ages.

For women who still want to work with Intermittent Fasting, there's a lot of hope left for you! Just make sure to follow these four steps to ensure that you're doing it in the most healthy way for your body and your future children. First, make sure you're very connected to your body. You'll want to be very aware if something on the inside seems "off" or "wrong" (bodily, emotionally, and mentally), especially considering all that's at stake, hormonally and reproductively.

Second, make serious effort to be aware of your body's cycles and note when things go askew. Without the right awareness of your menstruation, you risk going a long time with an altered cycle. This alteration might not sound like a lot, but it can affect many different aspects of your body and your childrearing potential.

Third, please don't try to combine strict dieting and Intermittent Fasting. I know you want to be fit and strong and slim, but you still want to make sure you're getting enough fat and calories, considering what your body is able to do with these right amounts of fat and calories.

Fourth and finally, make sure you're also not exercising too ferociously while you first transition to Intermittent Fasting. If you've been trying IF as a lifestyle for a while, you're welcome to add fitness and exercise back into the mix, but it is really dangerous for the female body to combine two intense practices at once. I understand the urge to lose weight and be healthy, but you'll need to make sure you're not eliminating *too much* from your body at any given time.

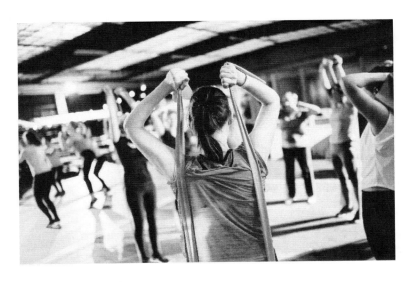

Given the complexity of the subject, I thought it was really useful to explain how Intermittent Fasting acts specifically on the female body. I dedicated a whole new book to it (*Intermittent Fasting for Women: Learn How You Can Use This Science to Support Your Hormones, Lose Weight, Enjoy Your Food, and Live a Healthy Life Without Suffering from Your Dietary Habits*)

If you're interested in the subject, I suggest you try to have a look at it. You can find the information <u>here!</u>

Chapter 5: For Some, Not Others

Given those potential complications concerning Intermittent Fasting, it is undeniable that it works perfectly for some, but not as well for others. This chapter will walk you through the body types and personality types that are well-suited for IF as well as those that are *definitely not* a good match. At the end of this section, you should know clearly whether or not IF is the next lifestyle choice for you.

5 Personality Types Perfect for IF

Some personality types are just perfectly matched for Intermittent Fasting, and 5 of them are included below.

1. <u>Sensitive introverts</u> are a great match for Intermittent Fasting. These types of people are often quiet and spend a lot of time alone, which means they're incidentally very in tune with the inner workings of their bodies and with the tendencies of their minds. By extension, therefore, these people will be extremely productive if they decide to try Intermittent Fasting because they'll be very aware of things going wrong almost immediately, but they'll also be very conscious of things going right.

2. <u>Problem solver</u> personalities will love the excitement provided by Intermittent Fasting! They'll see the problems posed by their bodies and their weight, and they'll be very eager to solve those problems with a combination of intelligence, cleverness, and bodily intuition. These people will meet the challenge of weight loss or boosting brain health with enthusiasm and

determination, knowing that a solution is in sight. They will be very likely to succeed in all IF endeavors.

3. <u>Health nut</u> personalities will love Intermittent Fasting for its interesting and divergent approach to body and mind health. They will love the long history of IF, as well as the words of assurance from great minds like Hippocrates, Paracelsus, and Benjamin Franklin. They will be devoted to the task of learning and perfecting IF in their lives based on all this appreciation, too, for they will know that learning and perfecting IF means they'll be learning more about and perfecting the self to be as healthy and vibrant as possible.

4. <u>Fitness experts</u> will love the potential Intermittent Fasting has to reinvent their bodies completely. They will appreciate the logic behind IF, too, in that it comes from the most primitive and ancient humans' survival expressions. They will see IF as a method of living out constant fitness, and they will be encouraged to approach their workouts differently, based on what they can achieve with restricted eating times. Furthermore, fitness experts will be highly intrigued by IF, which will make them willing to try things out—at least until things prove detrimental (which they will find, they won't).

5. <u>Confident and brave adventurers</u>, both in general and regarding food, will appreciate what Intermittent Fasting has to offer as well. These adventurers will recognize that change (of approach and focus) is almost always productive so that they will be drawn to the IF experience like flies to food! These types of people will try IF likely because they want to prove they can do it, but they'll stick with the strategy because they'll feel elated after their

bodies adjust to these odd and new eating times. They'll try it out for the adventure and stay for the blessings they receive.

5 Body Types Perfect for IF

Similarly, certain body types are spot-on in alignment with the goals and possibilities of Intermittent Fasting. 5 such body types are listed below.

1. <u>Heavy people</u> are bound to see huge successes in their attempts at Intermittent Fasting. As long as they can stay dedicated and committed to the eating and fasting time slots—and as long as they don't overeat during those eating windows—they should be able to see that fat almost melt away within weeks. In fact, heavy people who commit to Intermittent Fasting have the most to gain from their efforts, although they may have to add slight dieting or slight exercise to the mix to see these gains sooner.

2. <u>People with belly pudge</u> are also extremely well-suited to try Intermittent Fasting, for they should see results incredibly quickly. Just a bit of belly pudge mixed with a little less time spent eating each day can have a beautiful outcome, as long as the practitioner is dedicated and committed to his or her efforts. These types of people likely won't have to add diet or exercise to their routines to see that pudge disappear, but if they're interested in building muscle, they may have to add a little exercise after all.

3. <u>People with generally-fit bodies</u> pair well with the Intermittent Fasting lifestyle, too. These people are often already somewhat conscious of health, weight, and wellness. Additionally, they're often already conscious of how eating the right foods can act as a healing strategy for the body, mind, and soul. Therefore, these fit-bodied individuals won't have so much room to grow or change (bodily) with Intermittent Fasting, but they will find their mindsets and emotions changed in ways that are intriguing and lasting through this new lifestyle practice.

4. <u>People who are slim or heavy yet have trouble building muscle</u> are extremely well-suited to try Intermittent Fasting paired with light exercise. These types of people would do well with a method like 5:2 that requires five days of standard eating and exercise paired with two days in the week of fasting, wherein, for each day. No exercise is performed and only 500 calories are consumed. With the right alternation of eating and exercise with fasting and contemplation, these individuals are liable to see incredible growth of mind paired with an impressive loss of fat, favoring muscle.

5. <u>Women who are pear-shaped</u> have extra stores of body fat at the hips, tummy, and thighs, which makes them excellent candidates for great and lasting change through Intermittent Fasting! IF will help these women burn that fat into energy, and it will encourage their bodies to stop storing fat there in the future. With just a momentary recalibration through IF or a lifetime switch to the exercise, any pear-shaped woman can see those hips shrink down to a smaller size. With determination,

commitment, and practice, any bodily circumstances can change.

5 Personality Types that Don't Work

It might sound harsh, but some personality types aren't well-suited for the practice and lifestyle of Intermittent Fasting. If you relate to any of the 5 personality types below, make sure to do a lot of searching before you decide to try IF for yourself.

1. <u>Obsessive health or fitness experts</u> will definitely enjoy what Intermittent Fasting can do for them or their fitness-related clients, but these people are not encouraged to get dedicated to IF as a lifestyle, for they are bound to lose far too much. These people are only at risk with IF because their personalities are *obsessive* in nature. They won't be able to stop thinking about the fast, what it's doing for them, how to do it right, how to do it best, and how to be the best. These people are very likely to focus on the wrong parts of IF and turn it into an obsession rather than a healthy lifestyle. If anyone of this nature wants to try IF, I recommend they practice a little personality-softening (or ego-dampening) first.

2. <u>Compulsive athletes</u> are also potentially problematic about choosing Intermittent Fasting. If these types of people go the IF route, they're sure to see success, and they're sure to feel good, but it's very easy for compulsive athletes to push things *too far* for the sake of health or success. They can easily push way past their comfort zones without noticing, which is beneficial for sports, but it's not beneficial for one's body when the potential risk is one's health. For compulsive athletes who want to try IF

still, I recommend spontaneous skipping method. These people are invited to take on the less intense strategies like this one to experience what IF has to offer without losing themselves (and their health) in the process.

3. Overly-controlling people *might* enjoy Intermittent Fasting, but they could easily get too stuck in the details to fully appreciate what's happening. These people are liable to get too obsessed with perfection or with forcing the process to produce results (when they're not immediate or obvious). It's easy that they push themselves too fast and too hard to see results. Ultimately, these people can certainly grow, personality-wise, through Intermittent Fasting, but I'm concerned that their bodies might not benefit if their minds get the better of them. For those who qualify as overly-controlling and still want to try IF, just be patient with yourself as much as possible, and try not to force any of the processes.

4. Scatterbrained people and "space cadets" are similar to overly-controlling people when it comes to Intermittent Fasting because they can grow a lot through IF, personality-wise, but their main downfall is very different from that of overly-controlling people. Essentially, scatterbrained people or so-called "space cadets" often don't have the wherewithal to make sure they're sticking to schedules and following through on their IF timing goals. There's an obvious benefit to personalities like this, and some of my best friends qualify as "space cadets," but I'm not sure I'd recommend that they take on such a huge decision as trying IF—not unless they're truly ready to commit with full-force of body and mind.

5. <u>Overly-anxious or worrisome people</u> (as well as hypochondriacs) are not recommended to try Intermittent Fasting unless they're ready for some intense and serious personality work. These people are liable to get caught up in the details so much that they can't progress or move forward to be able to see real success with Intermittent Fasting. People who qualify as overly-anxious, worrisome, or hypochondriacs are still absolutely encouraged to *try* IF, but only as long as they're willing to work through the darkest parts of themselves first! Most people with these traits aren't ready for that, however, so I recommend they steer clear until they're emotionally and mentally better healed.

6 Body Types that Don't Work

Some body types, too, are simply not oriented to work well with Intermittent Fasting. It might not be what you want to hear, but if your body type correlates with any of the 6 below, you might want to take a step back and reevaluate before you decide to try IF.

1. <u>People with body dysphoria</u> are highly problematic candidates when it comes to Intermittent Fasting. These individuals receive false or skewed self-images through various means of perception, which means their sense of what's good about (or what needs to change about) themselves is absolutely off-kilter. These people may want to try IF even though they're beautifully fit and healthy. They may force themselves to try harsher IF methods because they don't feel like they're seeing the right results yet. People with body dysphoria are

encouraged to work on their self-image and accepting themselves before they try to change anything.

2. <u>People with eating disorders</u> are also incredibly problematic candidates for Intermittent Fasting. IF doesn't have to be practiced in unhealthy ways, and for the most part, it isn't. However, people with eating disorders (or with a history of them) will find that IF is an accidental gateway to a side of themselves that's not healthy whatsoever. People who are healing eating disorders are encouraged to try IF only with the verification from their doctors or nutritionists that this step is healthy and safe. Otherwise, wait a little while, heal yourself first, and then work on IF if your body can take it.

3. <u>Overly-thin people</u> probably don't need to try Intermittent Fasting at all. Most people apply IF to their lives to see weight loss, muscle building, or slimming progress. But people who are already very thin pose a threat to themselves and their health by adding IF to the mix. If you're already thin due to dieting, steer clear of IF. If you're thin due to exercise, cut the exercise if you want to try IF and make sure to keep eating the same number of calories! If you're thin due to genetics, it's debatable, but I still recommend you *not* try IF unless your doctor or nutritionist approves. You wouldn't want to do damage to yourself accidentally, would you!?

4. <u>People with severe diabetes</u> risk doing serious damage to their bodies and internal systems if they attempt Intermittent Fasting. If you severely have diabetes, IF might frustrate you because you won't be able to try it purely, and you will still have to take insulin throughout

the process. It's essential to note that you *won't be able to heal diabetes with IF*. If that's your goal, turn away right now. For those who just wanted to try IF to help the situation, you might be a little misled, too. People with severe diabetes should not try to restrict caloric intake seriously, they should not try to drink just liquids, and they should not try to fast for long periods; their bodies will not respond positively, and there are disastrous consequences. If people with severe diabetes still want to try IF, they're encouraged not to. Don't limit *when* you eat, eat healthier, more whole foods whenever possible.

5. <u>People with leaky gut</u> are not encouraged to turn to Intermittent Fasting to become healthier. In fact, people with leaky gut are often struggling to receive full nutrients from the foods they're actually consuming, so it's like they're on an IF lifestyle gone-wrong constantly, without even choosing it. Heal that leaky gut issue before trying IF, for the two together will put your body and health in a truly dangerous place.

6. <u>Pregnant & breastfeeding women</u> are not suggested to try Intermittent Fasting. There is much debate surrounding the issue of breastfeeding women, and it *can* be done safely, but for pregnant women, the case is not the same. The pregnant mother will be *unavoidably* providing nutrients to the child she's growing inside her, and if she restricts calories in any way, she will do damage to the fetus and its abilities to grow and develop. Divergently, breastfeeding mothers can supplement breastmilk with formula if things get tricky, and they can try less intensive IF methods to keep the breastmilk flowing well if they're really stuck to the idea of trying IF.

Chapter 6: The Many Faces of Intermittent Fasting

There are so many different ways to practice Intermittent Fasting that this entire chapter is dedicated to just those methods. I will walk you through 10 specific and different methods for IF before ending with a section on *how* to make your choice. By the end of this chapter, if you've chosen to try IF, you should feel that your IF plans have direction and form, and you should be excited to implement these new plans into your daily routine.

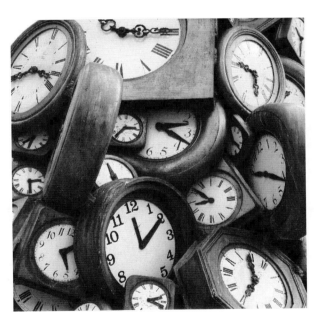

Explanation of Different Methods

Before you can start practicing Intermittent Fasting and incorporating it into your lifestyle, you'll have to know all the possibilities so you can choose the right one(s) for yourself, your goals, your habits, and your body/personality type. Read through the following 10 suggestions to find which methods sound most right to you.

Lean-Gains Method

The lean-gains method essentially focuses on the combined efforts of rigorous exercise, fasting, and a healthy diet. The fame surrounding this approach comes from its acclaimed success at turning fat directly into muscle. The goal is to fast within each day for 14-16 hours, starting when you wake up.

The ideal approach to lean-gains seems to be that you wake up and fast until 1 pm, doing some stretches and pre-workout warmups just before noon. Starting at noon, you would engage in training in whatever exercise you choose for an hour or less, ending with you breaking fast around 1 pm. Your meal at this time would be the largest of the day.

You would engage in your day as normal past then, as possible, eating again around 4 pm, then eating for the final time around 9 pm, giving yourself a ~15-hour fast until the next day at 1 pm. If you choose this approach yet feel a bit overwhelmed, you can work up to 15 hours, starting with a 13- or 14-hour fast only for the first week, building up to 15- or 16-hour fasting after that.

16:8 Method

16:8 method is one of the most popular methods among Intermittent Fasters. Essentially, you spend 16 hours within each day fasting, and the other 8 hours are your eating window. Most people try to choose their 8-hour eating window to be the times when they're primarily active. If you're a night person, feel free to make it a little later. Hold off eating during the daytime as much as possible then breakfast around 3 or 4 pm. For morning people, breakfast earlier, say, around 11 am, stopping food consumption by 7 pm.

16:8 is an incredibly flexible method that works for many different kinds of people. It's even flexible once you decide to try a particular fasting to eating window ratio. For example, if you don't seem to be jiving with the 11-7pm eating window, you can absolutely alter the next day to suit your needs better. Maybe try waiting until later in the day to breakfast! Try what you need to do, as long as you're keeping to that 16:8-hour ratio.

Whereas lean-gains method technically applies the same hourly ratio, it's much more strict regarding healthy diet and exercise regimen. 16:8 method does not need any type of exercise booster, but that's up to the practitioner. It is always best to try adding healthy dietary choices to one's IF eating schedule but don't try to restrict too many calories, as it can incorporate to feelings of lightheadedness and low energy. With 16:8, you can eat what you need and swap the hours around as desired.

14:10 Method

Similar to 16:8 method, 14:10 requires fasting and eating in varying degrees within each day. In this case, you would fast for 14 hours and engage in eating for a 10-hour window afterward. This method has the same flexibility as 16:8 in terms of what time of day it's arranged around, and how easy it is to troubleshoot. But it's additionally flexible in the sense that the eating window is two hours longer, accommodating people with more intense physical routines or daily demands, as well as people who simply need to eat a little later in the day to feel well.

20:4 Method

Whereas 14:10 method was an easier step *down* from 16:8 method, 20:4 method is definitely a step *up* in terms of difficulty. It's a more intense method certainly, for it requires 20 hours of fasting within each day with only a 4-hour eating window for the individual to gain all his or her nutrients and energy.

Most people who try this method end up having either one large meal with several snacks or they have two smaller meals with fewer snacks. 20:4 is flexible in that sense—the sense whereby the individual chooses how the eating window is divided amongst meals and snacks.

20:4 method is tricky, for many people instinctually over-eat during the eating window, but that's neither necessary nor is it healthy. People that choose 20:4 method should try to keep meal portions around the same size that they would normally have been without fasting. Experimenting on how many snacks are needed will be helpful as well with this method.

Many people end up working up to 20:4 from other methods, based on what their bodies can handle and what they're ready to attempt. Few start with 20:4, so if it's not working for you right away, please don't be too hard on yourself! Step it back to 16:8 and then see how soon you can get back to where you'd like to be.

The Warrior Method

The warrior method is quite similar to 20:4 method in that the individual fasts for 20 hours within each day and breaks fast for a 4-hour eating window. The difference is in the outlook and mindset of the practitioner, however. Essentially, the thought process behind warrior method is that, in ancient times, the hunter coming home from stalking prey or the warrior coming home from battle would really only get one meal each day. One meal would have to provide sustenance for the rest of the day, recuperative energy from the ordeal, and sustainable energy for the future.

Therefore, practitioners of warrior method are encouraged to have one large meal when they breakfast, and that meal should be jam-packed with fats, proteins, and carbs for the rest of the day (and for the days ahead). Just like with 20:4 method, however, it can sometimes be too intense for practitioners, and it's very easy to scale this one back in forcefulness by making up a method like 18:6 or 17:7. If it's not working, don't force it to work past two weeks, but do try to make it through a week to see if it's your stubbornness or if it's just a mismatch with the method.

12:12 Method

12:12 method is a little easier, along with the lines of 14:10, rather than 16:8 or 20:4. Beginners to Intermittent Fasting would do well to try this one right off the bat. Some people get 12 hours of sleep each night and can easily wake up from the fasting period, ready to engage with the eating window. Many people use this method in their lives without even knowing it.

To go about 12:12 method in your life, however, you'll want to be as purposeful about it as you can be. Make sure to be strict about your 12-hour cut-offs. Make sure it's working and feeling good in your body, and then you're invited to take things up a notch and try, say, 14:10 or maybe your own invention, like 15:11. As always, start with what works and then move up (or down) to what feels right (and even possibly *better*).

5:2 Method

5:2 method is popular among those who want to take things up a notch generally. Instead of fasting and eating within each day, these individuals take up a practice of fasting two whole days out of the week. The other 5 days are free to eat, exercise, or diet as desired, but those other two days (which can be consecutive or scattered throughout the week) must be strictly fasting days.

For those fasting days, it's not as if the individual can't eat anything altogether, however. In actuality, one is allowed to consume no more than 500 calories each day for this Intermittent Fasting method. I suppose these fasting days would be better referred to as "restricted-intake" days, for that is a more accurate description.

5:2 method is extremely rewarding, but it is also one of the more difficult ones to attempt. If you're having issues with this method, don't be afraid to experiment the next week with a method like 14:10 or 16:8, where you're fasting and eating within each day. If that works better for you, don't be ashamed to embrace it! However, if you're dedicated to having days "on" and days "off" with fasting and eating, there are other alternatives, too.

Eat-Stop-Eat (24-Hour) Method

The eat-stop-eat or 24-hour method is another option for people who want to have days "on" and "off" between fasting and eating. It's a little less intense than 5:2 method, and it's much more flexible for the individual, based on what he or she needs. For instance, if you need a literal 24-hour fast each week and that's it, you can do that. On the other hand, if you want a more flexible 5:2 method-type thing to happen, you can work with what you want and create a method surrounding those desires and goals.

The most successful approaches to the eat-stop-eat method have involved more strict dieting (or at the very least, cautious and healthy eating) during the 5 or 6 days when the individual engages in the week's free-eating window. For the individual to truly see success with weight loss, there will have to be some caloric restriction (or high nutrition focus) those 5 or 6 days, too, so that the body will have a version of consistency in health and nutrition content.

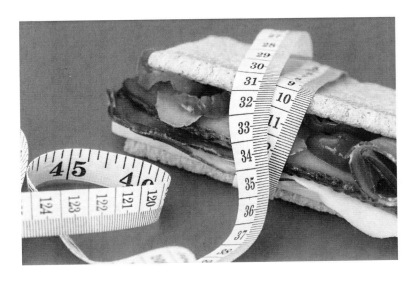

On the one or two days each week the individual decides to fast, there can still be highly-restricted caloric intake. As with 5:2 method, he or she can consume no more than 500 calories worth of food and drink during these fasting days so that the body can maintain energy flow and more.

If the individual engages in exercise, those workout days should absolutely be reserved for the 5 or 6 free-eating days. The same goes for 5:2 method. Try not to exercise (at least not excessively) on those days that are chosen for fasting. Your body will not appreciate the added stress when you're taking in so few calories. As always, you can choose to move up from eat-stop-eat to another method if this works easily and you're interested in something more. Furthermore, you can start with a strict 24-hour method and then move up to a more flexible eat-stop-eat approach! Do what feels right, and never be afraid to troubleshoot one method for the sake of choosing another.

Alternate-Day Method

The alternate-day method is similar to eat-stop-eat and 5:2 methods because it focuses on individual days "on" and "off" for fasting and eating. The difference for this method, in particular, is that it ends up being at least 2 days a week fasting, and sometimes, it can be as many as 4.

Some people follow very strict approaches to alternate-day method and literally fast every other day, only consuming 500 calories or less on those days designated for fasting. Some people, on the other hand, are much more flexible, and they tend to go for two days eating, one day fasting, two days eating, one day fasting, etc. The alternate-day method is even more flexible than eat-stop-eat in that sense, for it allows the individual to choose how he or she alternates between eating and fasting, based on what works for the body and mind the best.

The alternate-day method is like a step up from eat-stop-eat and 24-hour methods, especially if the individual truly alternates one-day fasting and the next day eating, etc. This more intense style of fasting works particularly well for people who are working on equally intense fitness regimens, surprisingly. People who are eating more calories a day than 2000 (which is true for a lot of bodybuilders and fitness buffs) will have more to gain from the alternate-day method, for you only have to cut back your eating on fasting days to about 25% of your standard caloric intake. Therefore, those fasting days can still provide solid nutritional support for fitness experts while helping them sculpt their bodies and maintain a new level of health.

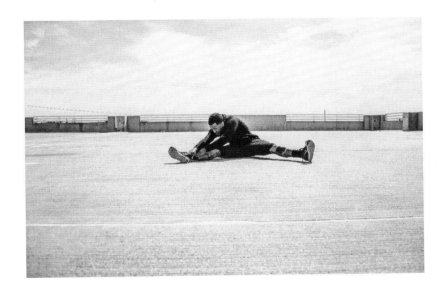

Spontaneous Skipping Method

Alternate-day method and eat-stop-eat method are certainly flexible in their approaches to when the individual fasts and when he or she eats. However, none of those mentioned above plans are quite as flexible as spontaneous skipping method. Spontaneous skipping method literally only requires that the individual skip meals within each day, whenever desired (and when it's sensed that the body can handle it).

Many people with more sensitive digestive systems or who practice more intense fitness regimens will start their experiences with IF through spontaneous skipping method before moving on to something more intensive. People who have very haphazard daily schedules or people who are around food a lot but forget to eat will benefit from this method, for it works well with chaotic schedules and unplanned energies.

Despite that chaotic and unorganized potential, spontaneous skipping method can also be more structured and organized, depending on what you make of it! For instance, someone desiring more structure can choose which meal each day they'd like to skip. Let's say he chooses to skip breakfast each day. Then, his spontaneous skipping method will be structured around making sure to skip breakfast (a.k.a.—not to eat until at least 12 pm) daily. Whatever you need to do to make this method work, try it! This method is made for experimentation and adventurousness.

Crescendo Method

The final method worth mentioning is crescendo method, which is very well-suited for female practitioners (since their anatomies can be so detrimentally sensitive to high-intensity fasts). Essentially, this approach is made for internal awareness, gentle introductions, and gradual additions, depending on what works and what doesn't. It's a very active, trial-and-error type of method.

Through crescendo method, the individual starts by only fasting 2 or 3 days a week, and on those fast days, it wouldn't be a very intense fast at all. In fact, it wouldn't even be so strict that the individual would have to consume no more than 500 calories, like with 5:2, eat-stop-eat, and others. Instead, these "fasting" days would be trial periods for methods like 12:12, 14:10, 16:8, or 20:4. The remaining 4 or 5 days out of the week would be open eating-window periods, but again, the practitioner is encouraged to maintain a healthy diet throughout the week.

Crescendo method works extremely well for female practitioners because it enables them to see how methods like 14:10 or 12:12 will affect their bodies without tying them to the method hook, line, and sinker. It allows them to see what each method does to their hormone levels, their menstruation tendencies, and their mood swings. Therefore, the crescendo method encourages these people to be more in touch with their bodies before moving too quickly into something that could do serious anatomical and hormonal damage.

Crescendo method will work extremely well for overweight or diabetic practitioners, too, for it will allow them to have these same "trial period" moments with all the methods before choosing what feels and works best, based on each individual situation.

Making Your Choice

When you make your choice from the 10 different options listed above, there are several things you'll want to keep in mind. First and foremost amongst those things will be the fact that you can always choose another method (or a more flexible one to start with) in case something doesn't work as you'd hoped. You can *always* troubleshoot your method in this way, and there's more on this topic in chapter 9 for those interested in troubleshooting (as well as for those being forced by their bodies to troubleshoot ASAP).

Ultimately, you'll also want to keep the following points in mind as you go about selecting your method: body type & abilities, lifestyle, daily tendencies, work routine, friends & family, and dietary choices. For all these considerations, remember what feels best to you, and remember to keep your goals with IF in mind at all times! If you ever feel like you're sacrificing your sanity or bodily health to attain these goals, go back to that step of troubleshooting, for you should never need to sacrifice those things to achieve any type of goals. Essentially, keep your eye on the prize and remember to choose what feels right and see what works from there.

<u>Consider your body type and abilities</u>. Think of how your body looks and feels and how much about it you'd like to change. Think about how you react to food and what it looks like when you're hungry. Think about those things you view as your "limits" and how comfortable you are with pushing. Are you a

fitness freak or a couch potato? Are you huskier or slimmer? Does your body hold onto fat or build muscle quickly? Do you retain water weight or not? Do you work out? Do you require a lot of water when you do? Consider all these things about your body and more, then compare them to the methods listed above. Compare them, too, to your overall goals with Intermittent Fasting to make sure that you're choosing a method that will help you actualize those goals as you conceive of them. If you're looking to lose weight quickly, try a method that works with days "on" and "off" between fasting and eating. If you're looking to build muscle, lean-gains method is probably the choice for you! If you're looking to boost your brain and heart, start with crescendo method and see where it takes you!

Consider your lifestyle. When do you normally wake up and how much sleep do you get on an average night? How hungry are you normally when you do wake up? How fast is your metabolism and when do you notice its peak? How do you make your living? Do you spend a lot of time in the car or on your feet or in an office? Are you constantly around other people or are you often alone? When you choose your method for Intermittent Fasting, make sure to consider all these lifestyle points. Maybe you wouldn't want to choose to time with a method that disallows you to eat when you normally need the most energy. Maybe you wouldn't want to choose a method that forces you to eat when you're supposed to be at work. Most of these methods have a degree of choice and flexibility, so when you do find one you like, remember that you don't have to put yourself in positions that go against your nature (or circadian rhythms) to achieve any of your goals. Stay flexible, keep your goals in mind, and respect the norms of your body!

Consider your daily tendencies. Do you eat mostly in the daylight hours or after the sun goes down? Do you go to work in the daytime or nighttime? Are you generally nocturnal, diurnal, or crepuscular? Do you have a lot of freedom and flexibility in your daily routines? Do you travel a lot for work? Do you spend a lot of time on the move? Do you have trouble remembering to eat? Are you the type of person that works out on the regular? Consider these themes in your life and more before you choose your method. Does it make sense for you to have low intake days where you consume 500 calories or less? Or does it make more sense for you to have extended periods in each day where you're just not eating based on your habits or tendencies or otherwise? Plan something that makes sense and respects your habits so that the transition into Intermittent Fasting is as easy and painless as possible.

Consider your work routine. Do you go to work in the morning or night? Are you allowed to eat at work? Do you work around food or in the food service industry? Do you work on your feet all day or by doing something strenuous? Do you receive purposeful or accidental exercise opportunities at work or are you just sitting in the same position all day? All these elements of your work routine will be important to consider as you decide which avenue of Intermittent Fasting to go down. You won't want to engage in a method like 20:4 if you're at work every day for incredibly short shifts. 20:4 works better for someone who works very long and distracting days. You won't want to try a method like 12:12 if part of your eating window involves being at work, when you're not allowed to eat at work. Remember to take your work life, routines, and restrictions into account when you go about making this choice, for you will make things much less harsh on yourself if you can look at this bigger picture from the beginning and planning stages.

Consider your friends, coworkers, and family. How loud are their opinions? Are their lives oriented toward health? Do they demean you a lot or make fun of your choices? Or are they encouraging all the time? Are these people your support system or are they your devils' advocates? Do you have the sense that they want to see you succeed? On the most basic level, are they nice to you and respectful of your choices? It might not seem that important, but the attitudes and supportive capacity of your friends, coworkers, and family can mean *the world* when you make a big choice like starting Intermittent Fasting in your life. Sometimes, people just don't want to see us succeed. They block our successes with jealousy, pride, ignorance, or arrogance. When friends and family act like this, it's better to choose a method that allows you to avoid discussing IF around them whatsoever. When friends and family are open and supportive, they shouldn't influence your choice that much at all; it's just when things are tenuous that you'll need to keep them (and your time around them) in consideration.

Finally, consider your dietary choices. Do you eat a lot of processed foods? Or do you eat a largely whole-foods, plant-based diet? Do you count calories? Do you cautiously skim nutrition facts? Are you looking for something specific like high fat, high fiber, or high protein? Are you hoping to change your diet entirely or are you trying to keep things the way they are? Are you willing to sacrifice items of your diet to actualize your goals? All these questions help determine which type of method you're going to be ready for. Essentially, if you're trying to change your diet entirely, a method with days "on" and days "off" will work best for you. In this case, try 5:2, alternate-day, eat-stop-eat, and spontaneous skip methods. However, if you don't want to change your diet that much at all, a method where you fast for periods within each day will be desirable instead.

Try methods like 20:4, 16:8, 14:10, or 12:12 for this type of situation.

As long as you make your selection with these 6 points in mind, you're sure to succeed with your Intermittent Fasting goals. You enable yourself to make the safest, smartest, best choice for your circumstances, and that's an incredible tool to use in so many different applications. In this case, it's a tool that will help keep you healthy, boost your brain, heal your heart, and shed that excess weight like melted butter!

As a reminder, your first choice still might not be the absolute *right one*, but by making the most educated choice possible, you're sure to start from a good place and learn a lot about yourself regardless. Make sure you have a runner-up method (or two!) that's easy to swap to just in case the first one doesn't seem to show progress. Work smarter, not harder! Plan ahead, do the research and know yourself. These are the truest steps to success that I know. And as always, don't be afraid to check with your doctor or nutritionist once the choice has been made. They'll be able to give you the final affirmation you need so you can get started on your new, healthy lifestyle with Intermittent Fasting in no time!

Chapter 7: Approaching Your Fast

It can be hard to transition into the first fasting period, but this chapter understand those struggles and comes equipped. Included in this chapter are 10 tips to getting started along with pointers on what to expect and what to look out for, and by the end, you should feel confident that your attempts at Intermittent Fasting will be productive, successful, and positive.

10 Tips to Get Started

Whether this is your first fast or your thousandth, everyone sometimes needs a little boost to get started. This section includes 10 tricks of the trade that will help you do just that.

1. Choose a method that aligns with your daily routine! When you work through chapter 6 and decide which method feels right, you don't have to choose something that's intentionally challenging. Go easy on yourself! Choose what feels like a natural extension of your daily routine. Your body, mind, and soul will thank you for it!

2. Plan your method! Don't go into your first Intermittent Fast (or yours fifth, for that matter!) without planning which method you'll choose, based on your lifestyle, routines, and tendencies.

3. Stick with your chosen method at least for the first week! You might feel tired of what you've chosen, and you might feel equally frustrated that things aren't working for you right away. But if you dedicate at *least* a week with a method, you can be sure whether or not it's helpful (and if not, you can discern how to tweak it to be better).

4. Do the research! If there's something else you've heard of (a rumor, a method, a fact, etc.) that are not included in this book, go find it! Research any questions that arise to be sure what you choose is right for *you*.

5. If you're unsure, check with your doctor or nutritionist! There are a lot of complexities involved with Intermittent Fasting, and one of the biggest complexities is the conundrum of your body. Your doctor or nutritionist will know your body and its needs best, so if you've decided on a method, run it by them to be sure that it's the one for you.

6. Alter your diet slightly ahead of time! If you're going to do a day-on, day-off style of fasting, start by cutting out snacks! Scale back what you're eating to make things easier on yourself when you start. On the other hand, if you're pairing diet with IF, start the diet *before* you start fasting so that you have a handle on that better (and so that you don't have to detox from certain foods while you're also fasting).

7. Check the nutrients you'll be receiving! Before you fast, make sure you're looking at the macronutrient levels of the foods you'll be eating. You want to make sure you have the right number of calories, carbs, proteins, and fats to stay healthy and energized.

8. Before the first day, make sure you're prepared! On the evening before your fast, make your dinner choice as conscious as possible, down to the timing. Don't gorge yourself and don't go crazy on something overly rich or decadent. Instead, eat a modest dinner that's not too late

and not *too* filling. Furthermore, don't snack after dinner so that you can wake up with a decent chunk of your fast already underway.

9. Keep a lot of drinks on hand! Drinks will be pivotal for keeping your energy and spirits up, so make sure you have them and that they're the *right* types of drinks to support IF! Check out chapter 8 for details in this respect.

10. To establish a routine, take things slow and don't be too hard on yourself! It can be hard to adjust to a whole new food-related lifestyle, so don't push yourself *too hard* too soon into the process. Stay realistic with your expectations for yourself and the fast.

What to Expect

When you start Intermittent Fasting, you'll want to keep several things in mind so that you know exactly what to expect. With these appropriate expectations in place, you'll have a much easier time troubleshooting your fast (see chapter 9) later on.

First, you'll want to expect mornings to be a whole new adventure. Sometimes, (based on the method you choose) your mornings will be slow and stagnant, and sometimes they'll be filled with energy. Sometimes, you may be super hungry in the morning, while other times you might be perfectly fine.

Second, expect that coffee will become your new best friend. Coffee will help you snap some energy when you're feeling low without food, and it can also keep you focused on something to do with your hands and mouth when you feel hungry but can't quite eat yet due to timing.

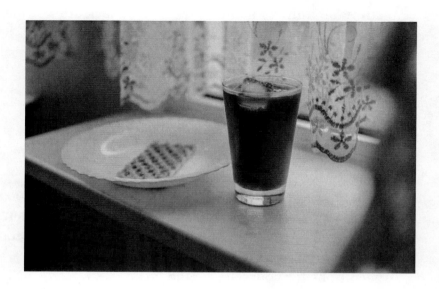

Third, expect that <u>your first week might be rough and moody</u>. You might have to build up a tolerance to all that Intermittent Fasting has to offer, but once you cross that first hurdle, you should have a much easier time moving on.

Fourth, <u>some things in your life will increase</u>. You'll become more present, more mindful, more conscious of the world and your feelings, and more conscious of how food makes you feel as well as what it makes you do and say.

Fifth, <u>some things in your life will decrease, namely your weight</u>! You could also see a decrease in sleep for the first few weeks, and while you go through the body's initial detoxification period, you might also find that your sleep isn't restful even when you can get it. Eventually, things will even out, and sleep will not be an issue anymore.

Sixth, <u>you will get cranky and emotional in the first few weeks</u>. During this period, you will be going through heavy detoxification of body and mind. You'll have to push through any anxiety, temper tantrums, and restlessness to keep your mind on the prize. You may even get a little smelly during this time as you sweat out all the bad, but your body and mind will thank you for this later!

Seventh, and finally, expect that <u>your relationship with food will completely change for the better</u>. You will be less of a slave to your cravings and desires, and you will be more understanding of people who live with less. You will be less dependent, more informed, more grateful, and less hangry when food takes a while.

While some of these expectations are relatively negative, most if not all have incredibly positive potential. Once you're through the first few weeks of your fast, you should see the silver lining of each expectation clearly.

What to Look Out For

All the above expectations should end up relatively resolved after the first week, but there will be signs in your body if things are *not* resolved and getting worse. These signs will be things to look out for, and if the situations don't improve with alteration and time, it may mean that IF isn't right for you after all. However, keep these tidbits in mind for your practice so that you can be on the lookout for your own best interest.

First, <u>watch out if you experience constant headaches, lightheadedness, or dizziness</u>. If you have these experiences just once or twice, that can be resolved, but if these arise *constantly*, there's a deeper problem that needs to be addressed.

Second, and furthermore, <u>if you're overly tired without the ability to sleep or constantly sleeping after the second week</u>, there's something wrong with your method or the way you're going about it.

Third, <u>watch out if you're getting hunger pangs that can't be dealt with</u>. Generally, during Intermittent Fasting, you'll experience hunger, and that's normal. You'll ride through the hunger wave and move past it. However, if these waves come again and again with no satiation, you might be in a bit of trouble. Check out chapter 10 for more details on this point.

Fourth, and finally, <u>watch for any severe personality changes</u>. If you start becoming obsessively compelled to practice your fast in new ways or if you feel that you're becoming overly controlling of or controlled *by* your fast, it might be time to take a break. Your personality can change, but if it does so in a way that aligns with the warnings mentioned in chapter 5, there's something to be concerned about.

These four points are all valid experiences to watch for, and if they appear without resolution, it may well be time to quit, but you can still try to troubleshoot your methods with the steps in chapter 9 before you make that call. As always, it's your body, so it's your choice. Just make sure it's the smartest and most informed choice you're capable of making.

Chapter 8: What to Eat/What Not to Eat

Before you start your first fast, however, it's helpful to know what's good to eat and drink versus what hurts the cause. This chapter is dedicated to that knowledge of what's good to eat and drink when Intermittent Fasting versus what to avoid at all costs.

10 Great Foods to Eat

When you're doing IF, you'll need to eat foods that give you enough energy to last until your next breakfast, and that can be tricky if you don't know what to look out for! This section lists 10 of the best foods to incorporate in your diet when practicing IF.

1. Avocado is high in calories and healthy fats, so it's perfect to have as a snack or in a meal.

2. Cruciferous vegetables like cauliflower, Brussel sprouts, broccoli, and more are full of fiber and so much more!

3. Potatoes of all kinds are great to satisfy one's hunger and provide a nutritional punch.

4. Legumes and beans of all varieties contain good carbohydrates that can help lower weight without too much restriction of calories.

5. Berries contain vitamin C, flavonoids, and antioxidants that will add a lot of good to your fast.

6. <u>Eggs</u> of any animal are packed with protein to help you build muscle and retain energy during the fast.

7. <u>Wild-caught fish</u> have a great amount of protein as well as vitamin D for one's brain and healthy fats and omega-3s for one's body.

8. <u>Anything high in protein</u> or <u>high in probiotic content</u> will be good to have along for the ride.

9. <u>Grains and nuts</u> are full of fiber, and healthy fats for snacks or meals during your fast's eating windows.

10. Spices such as <u>cayenne pepper, psyllium husk, or dried dandelion</u> are natural weight loss agents that can help anyone's process.

3 Foods to Avoid

On the flip side, some foods will absolutely set you back on your path to progress, and it will be equally important to know what to steer clear of. The following list includes three foods to avoid at all costs.

1. <u>Processed foods</u> will be the most important things to avoid, especially as you prepare for your fast.

2. <u>Highly GMO foods</u> are also things to avoid when you're working through your fast. They can offset the actual nutrition being provided by other foods in your diet.

3. <u>Sugary foods</u> may curb your appetite, but they won't do anything good for your body in the long run. Steer clear for your future ease.

10 Great Drinks

Even when you *are* fasting, drinks are still allowed! Make sure to choose drinks that are nutritious but not too filling, and mix it up whenever you can to keep things from getting stagnant for your taste buds (and body). 10 of the best drinks to incorporate for IF are listed below.

1. <u>Water with fruit or veggie slices</u> will provide nourishment and flavor for those times when you're fasting and need a little extra boost!

2. <u>Probiotic drinks</u> like kombucha or kefir will work to heal your gut and tide you over till the next eating window.

3. <u>Black coffee</u> will become your new best friend but be sure not to add cream and sugar! They detract from the good work coffee can do for your body during IF.

4. <u>Teas of any kind</u> are soothing as well as healing for various elements of the body, mind, and soul. Once again, be sure to omit the cream and sugar!

5. <u>Chilled or heated broths</u> made from vegetables, bone, or animals can sustain one's energy during times of fast, too.

6. <u>Apple Cider Vinegar shots</u> are great for the tummy and for healing overall! Hippocrates' remedy for any ailment

included this and a healthy regimen of fasting occasionally, so you're sure to succeed with this trick.

7. Water with salt can provide electrolytes, hydration, and brief sustenance for anyone whose stomachs won't stop grumbling.

8. Fresh-pressed juices are always great for the body, mind, and soul, and in times of IF, they can sustain one's energy and mood during day-long fast periods, in particular.

9. Wheatgrass shots are just as healthy as ACV shots, with a whole other subset of benefits. To awaken your body and give a jolt to your system, try these on for size.

10. Coconut water is more hydrating than standard water, and it's full of additional nutrients, too! Try this alternative if you need some enhancement to your usual water.

3 Drinks to Avoid

On the flip side, some drinks will definitely push you back from your goals, so keep an eye out for the 3 listed below! Avoid them at all costs.

1. Sodas of any kind, whether diet or non-diet, are to be avoided absolutely. They are high in sugar and riddled with terrible things for your body. Try to steer clear of this drink, especially during fast periods.

2. Coconut and almond drinks that are high in sugar are also to be avoided. Artificial sweeteners are killers for

one's blood sugar and insulin levels. They will reverse all the good work you've done, so be cautious.

3. <u>Alcohol</u> will distract you from your focus and commitment to the fast, and it will also steer your body off-course from where you want it to be. Try to IF soberly.

Chapter 9: Troubleshooting Your Fast

Sometimes, things don't go perfectly with Intermittent Fasting, but it's not hard to know what to correct when things do go down that problematic path. This chapter will lead you through troubleshooting techniques for your method, for your practice as a whole, and those sad moments when it might be time to stop. After reading this portion, you should feel safe and comforted by the knowledge that even *if* things don't work out well for you with Intermittent Fasting, there are several ways to turn things around.

5 Ways to Troubleshoot Your Method

For those times when you're not doing well, but you think the method's at fault, check in with these 5 tactics.

1. <u>Make sure your method relies on your body's natural rhythms</u>. If it does not, you will experience struggles and trials in your attempt to adjust to the lifestyle. To troubleshoot this issue, adjust your method of choice or change it entirely so that it lines up with your daily tendencies better.

2. <u>If you're constantly hungry on an alternate-day method (like 5:2), troubleshoot your process by switching to a daily method (like 16:8) instead</u>. You don't have to force yourself to fast for whole days with Intermittent Fasting! If it's not working for you, try something else like occasional eating windows each day.

3. <u>If you're feeling gorged after your eating windows but not *full*, there are a few things you can do</u>. Mainly, make sure

you're eating correctly each time you breakfast! You won't want to eat too quickly or too much, and these are the most common problems I've seen with IF. Eat a portion size you normally would and drink a sufficient amount of water with each meal or snack.

4. If you're getting dehydrated but still feeling okay, food- and health-wise, you might want to up the number of liquids you're taking in each day. Don't neglect liquids for the sake of focusing on food! Water, juices, teas, and more can help boost your goals, and they should never be forgotten.

5. Make sure your method of choice revolves around your work schedule, too! Especially if you work in the food industry, you'll want to plan your fasting times around periods when you know you won't be around (or tempted by) food. Spend your fasting periods in spaces that are safe, and spend this time doing things that are productive but not too strenuous. Your body and mind will thank you!

5 Ways to Pull it Back Together

On the other hand, sometimes it's not the method, it's the overall approach and strategy. In this section, you will find 5 ways to troubleshoot that avenue of the experience.

1. If you find yourself trying to force things to happen, take a step back and remember that there's only so much you can control! Your timing can only be *so* perfect, your training and exercise can only be *so* accurate, your body can only get strong *so* quickly, and your desires for

otherwise are just that—desires. Don't get caught up in imposed expectations, goals, or thoughts for timing or success. Take your experience day by day and let it reveal to you what it can. The less controlling and forceful thoughts you can have, the better.

2. If you find yourself trying to stop too eagerly, say within the first week or so, remember that there's really no reason to stop (especially within the first two weeks!) unless you're experiencing one of the three signs that it's truly time to stop (listed in the section just below this one). <u>Don't give up</u>! Push through any tension and anxieties, and if your concerns linger after the end of the second week, you're likely right that IF isn't the lifestyle choice for you. However, most will find that their systems get adjusted to IF perfectly after the end of the first week and that all concerns were truly for naught.

3. <u>If you find yourself losing inspiration, try to remember what motivated you to try Intermittent Fasting in the first place</u>! Go back to chapter 3 if you need and re-read all the potential benefits! Go back to the first medical case study you read that inspired you to try IF—or talk to the person that recommended the lifestyle of IF to you. By getting back in touch with these inspirational roots, your experience will be made all the better.

4. If you find yourself getting stuck on worries or concerns for your safety, <u>remember to stay grounded in your body</u>! Don't get so excitable that you're stuck in your head, thinking the worst about things that aren't even happening to you! If you find yourself falling into these patterns of anxiety, remember to try thinking past and through these trials. On the other side, you will

remember *why* you tried IF, *what good* it can do for you, and *how good* your body is already feeling because of it.

5. <u>If you find your path blocked by unappreciative or unaccepting family or friends, it might be time to get some distance from them</u>. You can reclaim your choices in life by making them purposefully in front of these people or consciously and contemplatively on your own, away from them. Based on how intense these family members' and friends' opinions are, you can choose to avoid these people entirely, you can choose not to talk IF themes with them, or you can simply choose not to fast or breakfast around them. There are many ways to reclaim your process in instances such as this; you'll just need to remember your purpose and stand your ground (for yourself).

3 Signs it is Time to Stop

Sometimes, it's not the approach, and it's not the method either. Sometimes, it's just time to call it quits, and it's not so much about quitting as it is about saving your body. If any of the following 3 signs come up, it's probably best to stop.

1. <u>If any of your health struggles have gotten worse despite your attempts with IF, it might be time to stop</u>. Especially if you've troubleshot your plan, tried to turn it around and received no betterment to your situation, it's probably time for you to stop IF for good.

2. <u>If you experience intense burning in the pit of your stomach or pains inside your chest cavity, despite having tried to troubleshoot your method, it could be that IF is</u>

causing more problems for you than it's healing. With these dangerous pains in place, stop IF and discuss these issues with your doctor or a nutritionist.

3. If you vomit uncontrollably despite having eaten nothing or if you have diarrhea that's almost constant, you're not going about this right. For now, just stop trying IF and discuss what's going on with your doctor or nutritionist. They will likely be able to reveal what's going wrong with your process—otherwise, it's just plain time to stop.

Chapter 10: Am I Hungry? Or Am I Starving?

One of the most confusing elements of Intermittent Fasting (especially for beginners) is how to tell when you're just hungry versus when you're in danger of starving. This chapter will lead you through several tips to control your hunger, signs of starvation, and ways to pull everything back together if starvation takes hold over hunger.

5 Tips to Control Hunger

If you can tell you're just hungry, use one of the 5 tips to counteract that belly grumble!

1. First things first, you *will* encounter hunger quite a lot. You will come to build a new relationship with hunger altogether, and you will know it as its unique feeling that's different from starvation entirely. With these feelings of hunger, it's best to <u>think of it as a wave passing through you that you can ride</u>. Once you ride the wave, it will pass and return in time, but you will teach yourself patience, stamina, and endurance by practicing this visualization for yourself.

2. If you experience occasional dizziness or lightheadedness, you're likely feeling the effects of low blood pressure or low blood volume. You can heal this lowness yourself by <u>drinking water with just a pinch of salt to restore your system's electrolytes</u>. You could also try taking magnesium supplements to correct these sensations. Remember, constant feelings of this sort are signs to stop, but occasional states like this are normal.

3. When your stomach starts to grumble literally, <u>don't be alarmed</u>! Your stomach is just working out the last bits inside it to send along to your intestinal system. These grumbles are totally natural and utterly normal. Ride through the grumbly waves just like you would for the sensation of hunger, and your stomach will stop doing its thing in just a few minutes, most likely.

4. <u>Some people experience hunger as a variety of moodiness</u>. If you tend to get "hangry" or sassy when you're hungry, there are a couple of things you can do. The most obnoxious method to deal with feelings like this is just to see if it lingers after you're fully adjusted to IF as a lifestyle. If you start feeling moody on top of being hungry, you can also choose the subtle method, which is to get introspective with yourself and try to figure out how to best these feelings for the sake of your health and growth. Essentially, if you're feeling sassy, hangry, or moody, these emotions are signs of pure hunger. They're not to be fearful of, and they're easy to troubleshoot. All you need to do is bear through it and try to be better.

5. <u>Alternate coffee and water</u> as your chosen drinks during fast periods! Yes, you're going to be hungry. Yes, you're going to want to eat. However, you're going to need to stay strong and consistently supplement foods with drinks during these fasting periods. As your right-hand-guys (drink-wise), keep coffee and water at your side constantly and make sure to alternate between the two! Just coffee will keep you hungrier more often, and just water will make you feel utterly empty without any energy. By switching between the two, you'll help your body deal with hunger in big ways.

5 Signs of Starvation

If it feels like more than just hunger, check in with these 5 signs to ensure you're not on the path to starvation.

1. The first sign of starvation mode (or the state of metabolic damage) is that <u>your brain can't handle functions that were considered "normal" before IF</u>. If you find your cognitive skills significantly decreased, your approach to IF is not benefitting you. You should be able to experience sharper and more purposeful cognition through the addition of IF. The opposite is absolutely a warning sign.

2. Another sign of your body going into starvation mode will be <u>inconsistent or consistently low energy levels</u>. For the individual experiencing the early stages of starvation, there will be intense mood and energy drops that distract from the focus and energy going into his or her day. There could also be almost constant periods of very low energy that are detrimental to the individual's day.

3. Another sign that your body might be headed in this direction would be the <u>intense and noted loss of weight with nothing gained back</u> in terms of muscle, despite exercise and intermittent food intake. Yes, you certainly *want to* lose weight, but there are many ways of losing weight that is healthy (in relation to IF) yet losing an excessive amount in a very short period is *not* that healthy way.

4. A couple more bodily signs of starvation mode involve <u>excessive bloating or gas, heartburn or reflux, fluid</u>

retention in ankles, weight *gain*, loss of muscle mass, completely ceased menstruation in women, decreased immunity (or longer flu and cold periods), or severe sleep disturbances. Anyone of these signs is troubling alone, but when two or more are experienced together, you can be *sure* you're in a state of metabolic damage.

5. A few final mental and emotional signs of starvation mode include severe mood swings, a prevalence of depression or anxiety (especially where there was none before IF), lowered libido, seriously lowered energy, or lack of interest in living. Any of these signs alone is detrimental enough to warrant concern, so if any of these experiences arise for you, it may be time to stop IF for good.

3 More Ways to Pull it Back Together

Once you're able to tell the level of threat you're at (if it's hunger or truly starvation), there are other ways to pull things back together and get the practice going once more. 3 of those approaches are listed below.

1. If you've troubleshoot your hunger, and you're ready to go back for more, think harder about what snacks and meals you're eating when you breakfast! You can eat highly-nourishing, calorie-dense foods that have healthy fats and all the proteins your body could need. Don't neglect your responsibilities along with that ability! It's up to *you* to choose the healthy options and to purposefully feed yourself with living, healing foods.

2. For those who get too close to (or too deep into) starvation mode, you can <u>bring things back together by taking a few days off of the fast entirely</u>. Take a break and come back to things with a refreshed mind and reinvented plan of attack. With a new method and mental approach—as well as the unfortunate experience of starvation—your IF adventure can be completely re-engaged for the better.

3. If you've struggled with hunger and starvation, you might be able to practice your version of IF that isn't listed in chapter 6 in this book at all. <u>Based on your body and your experience, you may be able to completely invent your own, holistic approach to IF</u> that no one else has ever thought of before. Perhaps your approach needs certain timing in each day to work. Perhaps it requires certain foods and not others. Perhaps it requires the support of others and a specific setting. Perhaps it needs the right mindfulness to not lead to starvation. Whatever they happen to be, with your failures under your belt, you will learn what works for you and what doesn't, which gives you the unique opportunity to invent your Intermittent Fast from scratch to incorporate the complexities of your experience. Embrace that potential and try again if you're able!

Chapter 11: Flavors of Fasting

Intermittent Fasting is great for the body, mind, and soul for a variety of reasons. This chapter shows the many different applications of Intermittent Fasting. For example, it can be productive for weight loss, heart health, brain health, depression, and so much more, and this chapter will give you those inside scoops.

Fasting for Weight Loss

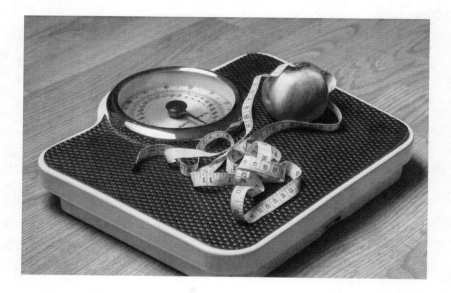

For the body, Intermittent Fasting works magic with weight loss. By eating less, eating less often, or eating more consciously, practitioners restrict their intake of calories, which is almost guaranteed to have weight loss effects in the body. For the practitioner fasting 15 hours a day, there's a trajected loss of about 3 pounds of fat each week. That's without any attempt at dieting or exercise. When it comes down to it, Intermittent Fasting is positively correlated with weight loss 100% of the time. Give it a try to get rid of that pesky belly fat! You'll be so glad you did—as long as you're up to the commitment!

Fasting for Diabetes

For the body and mind, Intermittent Fasting is helpful about those with Types 1 or 2 diabetes. A low-intensity approach to IF will enable the individual with diabetes to experience more consistent energy levels, more glucose absorption into the cells, and more weight loss that's productive than ever before. To be clear, IF is not a cure for diabetes, and it does still pose some issues, but as long as the practice is low-intensity and taken with care, the individual is sure to see significant growth of both body and mind.

Fasting for Heart Health

Just like with diabetes, Intermittent Fasting doesn't cure heart disease, but it can definitely make things better! In specific, relating to heart health, IF can enable the body to have lower blood pressure, lower cholesterol levels, less triglycerides, and fewer instances of inflammation. All of which contribute to heart disease (and worse). Anyone dealing with heart struggles is invited to try IF, for it can reverse potentially disastrous circumstances with just a few lifestyle changes.

Fasting for Brain Health

Intermittent Fasting can do incredible things for one's brain. It's crazy to think that people dealing with mental struggles of dementia, Alzheimer's, and more can have their situations eased with consistent periods of low caloric intake! It's even crazier once you know *how* IF helps these individuals. In specific, IF can cause the literal growth of new brain cells, and it can make one's cognition heightened even in times of distress. It can increase neuroplasticity overall, and it can help the brain & body learn how to burn fat for fuel in addition to just sugar (which is the main issue for people with diabetes!). Fat burns cleaner and more efficiently as fuel for the body and brain. Finally, IF can also give a gigantic boost to one's energy levels, which easily relates to one's brain power. Try Intermittent Fasting for your body, and you'll be elated to see what also can happen in your brain!

Fasting in Medicine

Fasting has been used for medical reasons for decades, too, and those medical reasons are extremely varied! Even today, before a routine surgery, your surgeon will tell you not to eat or drink anything past a certain hour. Before a serious check-up requiring intensive procedures, your doctor might ask you to do the same. Even before our pets go to get surgeries, their veterinarians will ask we not feed them past a certain time. Then there are the words of Hippocrates and Paracelsus (among others) from ancient Greece, both of whom advocated for fasting to enact medical health. From ages across time to today, fasting has been used to further medical procedures and to encourage overall healing for patients with a variety of conditions.

Fasting for Cancer

There are so many benefits of Intermittent Fasting, but none are so profound as its abilities to aid cancer patients. Recent studies have proven that IF both decreases cancer regrowth rates, as well as the risk of cancer in individual practitioners. These effects are most often related to IF's abilities to lower glucose production, to boost the creation of tumor-killing cells, to rebuild the immune system and each cell at a time, and to balance one's nutritional consumption. Altogether, these effects work wonders for people battling life's most terrifying disease.

Fasting for Depression

While Intermittent Fasting can have such healing effects on body, mind, and soul that cancer symptoms are lessened in intensity or erased in entirety, it also has the same three-fold effects for individuals battling depression. The World Health Organization has stated that depression is on the rise across the globe, yet its symptoms and effects on the body, mind, and soul are so various that it's hard to tackle any one element at a time. Thankfully, Intermittent Fasting addresses many elements at once, healing all of them in kind. IF's effects on hormone production throughout the body have sensational consequences that align with increased mood, lessened anxiety, and a greater sense of well-being and purpose.

Chapter 12: Q & A

To wrap things up before our final chapter of recipes, this section is all about those final questions that might linger in your mind. It's about addressing your concerns and putting your mind at ease. If you have a question that doesn't appear to be answered anywhere in this book, ask to your trusted nutritionist and make sure to do things right.

15 Questions & Answers about IF

Whether they're about methods, strategies, approaches, measurements of success, or otherwise, these questions (and their respective answers) should address any lingering concerns or confusions for any future (or current) IF practitioners.

1. Who is Intermittent Fasting for?

   IF is actually for anyone! It works best for people who are simply serious about making their health better and about changing their weights for the better without sacrificing their diets.

2. What should I consider before my first fast?

   Think of your bodily limitations, your daily routine, your work schedule, and your tendencies with hunger and thirst. The more you know about yourself, the better! On the other hand, the more you know about the method you're going to try, the better, too! Consider every detail you can, from your personality to your body weight, your tendencies, your cravings, and more. Together, all these details will help you make your first fast the best and most lasting change in your life.

3. If I'm diabetic, should I try IF?

    Absolutely! Give IF a try, but don't be too strict with diet or exercise while you attempt it. Additionally, don't be too strict with your timing or snack restriction. Diabetic individuals can experience troubles with IF when they limit themselves too much, so make sure you're not sacrificing your health but definitely give it a try!

4. Will IF help with more than weight loss?

    Yes, definitely! Intermittent Fasting can heal the brain, the heart, the digestive system, the mood, and so much more! It's not just about weight loss, and anyone who insists it is just lying to you.

5. Which method of IF is best?

    The answer to this question is more subjective than objective. There's no one method that's best for everyone. In fact, each individual should choose the method that works best for him or her based on the guidelines listed in chapter 6.

6. Where should I begin if I'm interested in IF?

    Start by doing some reading! Research IF and see what it can do for you. Then, start making the simple steps to your own IF transition. These simple steps include snacking less, eating less often late at night, waiting a little longer to eat in the morning, and making sure to eat dinner a little bit earlier.

7. I'm breastfeeding—should I try IF or wait until I'm done?

Great question! Generally, I suggest you waiting until you're done breastfeeding to try IF or to reinstate it again. While you're breastfeeding, your body needs a specific subset of nutrients to produce what your baby needs. With an intense exercise regimen and practice of caloric restriction, you may do more harm to your body and your baby than good. It's not worth the risk, but as I wrote above, there's a possibility. For more details, check my other book *Intermittent Fasting for Women: Learn How You Can Use This Science to Support Your Hormones, Lose Weight, Enjoy Your Food, and Live a Healthy Life Without Suffering from Your Dietary Habits*

8. Should I exercise while I try IF?

As you transition into IF, start by trying to exercise occasionally, but don't expect that you'll be able to exercise as much as you had been without IF. Start small and build up to see what your body can handle, given the restricted intake. Women and diabetic individuals are almost exclusively recommended to *not* exercise while attempting IF. The consequences are too problematic for me to want you to push those boundaries.

9. Should I diet while I try IF?

You can certainly try! However, most people will realize that strict dieting does *not* pair all that well with IF unless it's the Keto Diet. People who diet by calorie counting will *not* benefit by taking this strategy into IF. People who diet by restricting protein or fat will equally *not* benefit with IF. Therefore, if you *do* combine dieting and IF, make sure your diet isn't too strict, and leave wiggle room for growth and troubleshooting. If you're attempting the Keto Diet, with its helpful divisions of fat, protein, and carbs, you may find that your diet is perfect for IF. As always, take things one day at a time, and don't cling too harshly to your diet! There may be times when it helps, but there will be times when it doesn't. Just stay open to changes and fluctuations in your experience.

10. I'm working on IF right now—why do I have a headache constantly?

Not everyone feels this type of head pain while fasting, but it is more often women than men that go through this experience. Due to studies done on Islamic peoples observing Ramadan, we can tell that the cause to this pain is not always dehydration. In fact, it's much more related to the kind of headache one gets after quitting coffee drinking. Essentially, it's a withdrawal symptom from something, and it *will* fade and go away after you keep practicing the fast. If it doesn't go away, it might be time to stop (see chapter 9).

11. Is it okay to drink during IF or is it strictly no intake?

It's absolutely acceptable (and even recommended!) for individuals to drink during fast periods. Just try to make sure your drink has no calories (so no soda, not a lot of juice, etc.), and you should be aligned with your goals! Simply remember that fasting periods are supposed to be times of rest for your body and mind, so you won't want to add anything too intense to that bodily mix in these moments. Keep the calories of the drink low, and you'll be set.

12. If I take supplements and vitamins each day, should I stop them while trying IF?

The short answer to this question is yes. The longer answer to this question is that you might want to hold off on taking your supplements on days when you're fully fasting. However, if you're not doing day-on, day-off fasts but fasting and eating within each day instead, you should have no problem continuing to take all supplements daily, as you normally would.

13. Will IF screw up my metabolism?

Your metabolism is much more connected to your body fat than most people know and are taught. Therefore, all concerns over messing up one's metabolism through IF are largely unfounded. The truth is that as your body fat goes down, so will your metabolism. The less you have to burn, the less intensely your metabolism works, but that's all balanced out by the body's natural processes. Essentially, there's no way you can screw this up.

14. Is IF safe for pregnant women and expecting mothers?

Many different groups hotly debates this, but the gist of the answer is that it depends on the mother, the situation, and the advice of the mother's doctor. Sometimes, IF poses no threat, while other times it's disastrous. Err on the side of caution and speak with your doctor or nutritionist first.

15. I have hypothyroid. Should I try IF or not?

With hypothyroid, you should still be able to try IF! The trick for you will be to make sure you never fast for more than a day at a time. Your bodily rhythms will be greatly distressed if you attempt to fast more than 24 hours at once.

Chapter 13: 15 Recipes for IF on the Keto Diet

For this recipe portion, I've mixed the Keto Diet in with our attempts for Intermittent Fasting because the two pairs so easily. Typically, the Keto Diet is divided into the following nutritional percentages: around 70% of calories from fat, around 20% of calories from protein (a moderate amount), and no more than 10% of calories from carbohydrates.

The main focus of the Keto Diet is to remove excess carbohydrates from one's diet to enable the increased production of ketones in the body, which are essentially molecules that produce fuel for the individual. With less glucose, or blood sugar, in the body (resulting from that restriction of carbohydrates), the liver breaks down fat cells and produces ketones instead. Therefore, the body runs mostly off fat and burns fat more consistently because fat becomes *essential* for its ability to breakdown into ketones (a.k.a.—energy for brain and body).

With this increased production of ketones, the body becomes slimmer and fit, less bulked with fat, less sugar-crazed, and more energized even if the individual is intermittently fasting as well. In fact, Intermittent Fasting increases the body's production of ketones differently (by producing ketosis, a fruitful metabolic state), so the two pair well together in that ketonic connection.

As a general warning, just like with Intermittent Fasting, some body types will not do well with this type of metabolic shift. If you are diabetic, breastfeeding, or taking medication for high blood pressure and you still want to attempt Intermittent

Fasting, I do not recommend adding the Keto Diet to the mix. For the rest of my readers, this section should help to solidify those weight loss and lifestyle goals in no time.

Breakfasts

Low-carb breakfasts might seem counter-intuitive, but they're not only just possible! They're also delicious, nutritious, and packed with productive energy. Whichever of the two recipes below you choose, your mornings are sure to give you exactly the boost you need, and if you need more options, there are surely other sources at your disposal.

Frittata with Spinach and Mushrooms

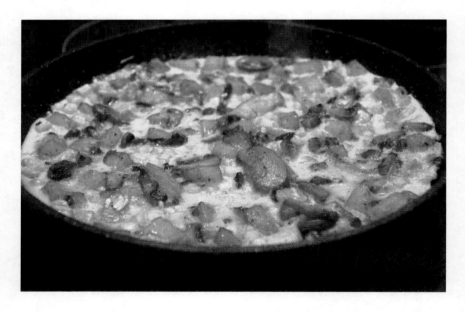

Tasty, simple, and packed with nutrition, this breakfast is best for sharing with a group of people (so there are no leftovers!) to get your day started.

This recipe needs 10 minutes of prep and about 35 minutes of cooking. It will make 4 helpings.

- Fat—59 g

- Protein—27 g
- Net Carbs—4.1 g
- Calories—661

What to Use:

- Butter (2 tablespoons)
- Bacon (6 ounces, coarsely diced)
- Spinach (8 ounces)
- Eggs (8, large-sized)
- Heavy Cream (1 cup)
- Shredded Cheese (6 ounces)
- Salt & Pepper (to taste)

What to Do:

- Start by heating the oven to 350 degrees while bringing the 2 tablespoons of butter to medium heat in a frying pan on the stovetop.
- When heated, add bacon to pan and cook until desired crispiness. Then add the spinach and stir together until soft. Remove both from pan and drain the fat. Set to the side for now.
- In a separate medium-sized bowl, combine the eggs and cream. Once whisked together, grease a 9x9 baking dish and pour the mixture in.
- Stir in bacon, spinach, and any shredded cheese. Put dish and mixture in the oven.
- Bake 30 minutes until perfectly browned.

Pancakes with Berries

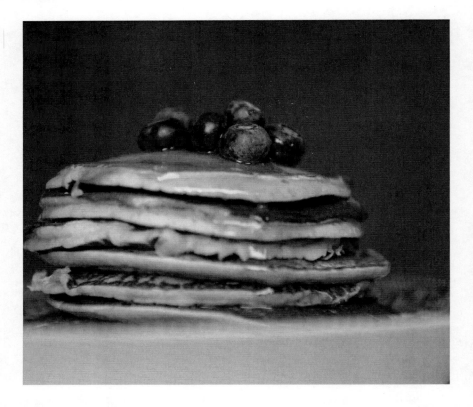

"How do you make low-carb pancakes?!" you might be asking yourself, and the answer is just within reach! These pancakes have a unique flavor, but they're nutritionally amazing and great for starting your day.

This recipe needs 5-10 minutes of prep and about 20 minutes of cooking. It will make 4 helpings.

- Fat—39 g
- Protein—13 g
- Net Carbs—5 g
- Calories—425

What to Use:

- Eggs (4, large-sized)
- Cottage Cheese (7 ounces)
- Psyllium Husk Powder (1 tablespoon)
- Butter or Coconut Oil (2 ounces)
- Berries (0.5 cup, for topping)

What to Do:

- In a medium-sized mixing bowl, stir together the first three ingredients and let sit. After about 10 minutes, the mixture should be perfectly thickened.
- Grab a large-sized non-stick skillet and heat butter or coconut oil until melted. Portion out 0.5-cup scoops of the batter onto the skillet and cook 4 minutes on each side until done.
- Prepare berries as desired (sliced or whole, etc.), and top finished pancakes with them for a delightful boost of sweetness.

Lunch

For lunch, let's not do something too big or too packed with sugar. Salads, half-wraps, stir-fries, and chicken salads will do just fine! Regardless of your tastes, there should be something to suit your pallet in this section. Given your goals and vision for Intermittent Fasting, you're bound to see progress with these recipes in no time.

Pulled Pork Sliders

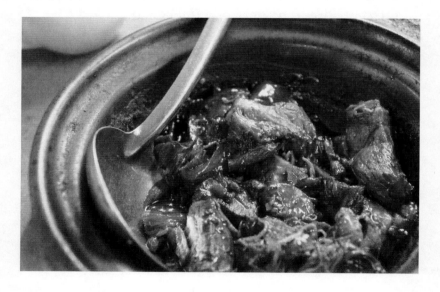

With its homemade sauce and perfect tenderness, this slider will make you feel gleeful and packed with energy to keep your intermittent fast going strong for the rest of the day.

This recipe needs 20 minutes of prep and about 45 minutes of cooking. It will make 4 helpings.

- Fat—15.1 g
- Protein—9.1 g

- Net Carbs—3.6 g
- Calories—184

What to Use:

- Pork Roast (3 pounds, boneless, cut into inch pieces)
- Butter (1 tablespoon)
- Salt (2 teaspoons)
- Garlic Powder (2 teaspoons)
- Onion Powder (1 teaspoon)
- Black Pepper (1 teaspoon)
- Smoked Paprika (1 tablespoon)
- Tomato Paste (2 tablespoons)
- Apple Cider Vinegar (0.5 cup)
- Coconut Aminos (2 tablespoons)
- Bone Broth (0.5 cup)
- Butter (0.25 cup, melted)

What to Do:

- Trim any fat from your pork roast and then cut it into appropriate chunks.
- In a small-sized bowl, combine salt, paprika, pepper, onion and garlic powders and then rub the mixture onto the pork.
- Grab a large-sized skillet and melt the tablespoon of butter before adding your chunks of pork to the skillet as well.
- In a separate, medium-sized bowl, combine all other ingredients and pour over the pork in the skillet.
- Boil the mixture to start then simmer for 30 minutes until meat is tender and is easy to pull apart in the sauce.
- Serve on low-carb bread alternative or eat in portions alone.

Curry Chicken Half-Wraps

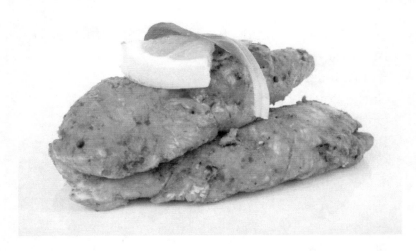

With a little effort, these half-wraps can be substituted for lettuce wraps, but they're just as delicious either way! Have as many as you need to keep that energy up throughout your day. There is a little less fat in this recipe than there could be, but you can correct that (as you like) by adding a little more cream as your garnish, or you could add a sprinkle of feta cheese on top, too.

This recipe needs 5 minutes of prep and about 20 minutes of cooking. It will make 2 helpings.

- Fat—36.4 g
- Protein—50.9 g
- Net Carbs—7.2 g
- Calories—554

What to Use:

- Chicken Thighs (1 pound, boneless & skinless)

- Onion (0.25 cup, minced)
- Garlic (2 cloves, minced)
- Curry Powder (2 teaspoons)
- Salt (1.5 teaspoons)
- Butter (3 tablespoons)
- Cauliflower Rice (1 cup)
- Low-Carb Wraps (cut into halves)
  - Or lettuce leaves
- Yogurt or Sour Cream (0.25 cup, for garnish)

What to Do:

- Start by preparing your chicken thighs; cut them into one-inch pieces.
- Take a large-sized skillet and heat 2 of the 3 tablespoons of butter on the skillet at medium heat. Add onion and cook till soft and browned.
- Stir in chicken pieces, garlic, and salt. Cook for about 10 minutes.
- Stir in the last tablespoon of butter, curry powder, and cauliflower rice. Cook about 5 minutes longer.
- Serve in lettuce leaves or half-wraps, and top with a scoop of cream! Enjoy.

Sautéed Mushrooms & Bacon with Greens

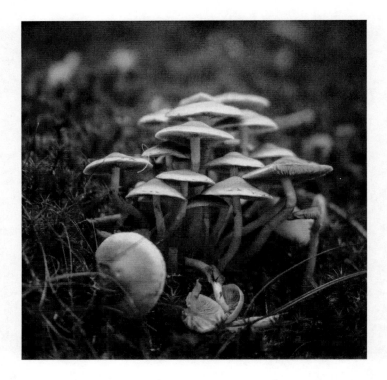

With a modest side-salad, this entrée is both elegant and appropriately filling. You'll want to bring it out when friends come around—or even for date night! The possibilities are endless.

This recipe needs 10 minutes of prep and about 10 minutes of cooking. It will make 2 helpings.

- Fat—14 g
- Protein—15 g
- Net Carbs—8.4 g
- Calories—257

What to Use:

- Bacon (4 slices, cut into half-inch pieces)
- Mushrooms (2 cups, halved; your choice)
- Salt (0.5 teaspoon)
- Thyme (2 sprigs fresh herb, destemmed)
- Garlic (3 cloves, minced)
- Greens (2 cups; your choice)
- Salad Dressing (0.25 cup; your choice)

What to Do:

- Assemble the side-salad quickly by taking your choice of greens and sprinkling on a bit of dressing. Set aside or place in the refrigerator for just a few moments.
- Take a large-sized skillet and bring to medium heat. Add bacon and cook until desired crispiness is reached. Stir in mushrooms and bring to browned color.
- Stir in salt, thyme leaves, and garlic. Cook 5 minutes then serve hot alongside your salad.

Easy Chicken Salad

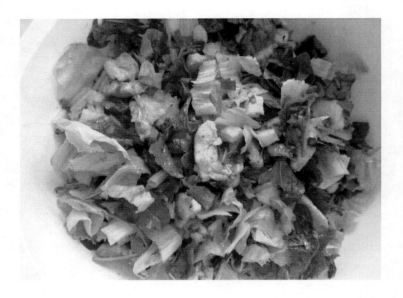

With a bread substitute of your choosing or over greens, this chicken salad will do just the trick. It even adds an interesting flavor spin on the traditional chicken salad that you can either appreciate or alter to your preferences. There is a little less fat in this recipe than what is typical of the Keto Diet, and you can correct that (for your liking) by adding more mayo or a bit of cheese to your salad as well.

This recipe needs 1 hour and 30 minutes of prep and about 15 minutes of cooking. It will make 6 helpings.

- Fat—19 g
- Protein—24.8 g
- Net Carbs—1.1 g
- Calories—279

What to Use:

- Chicken Breast (1.5 pound)

- Celery (3 stalks, sliced)
- Mayo (0.5 cup)
- Brown Mustard (2 teaspoons)
- Salt (0.5 teaspoon)
- Dill (2 tablespoons, fresh & chopped)
- Pecans (0.25 cup, chopped)

What to Do:

- Heat the oven to 425 degrees and line a baking sheet with parchment paper, aluminum foil, or baking spray.
- Add chicken breast and cook until done throughout. This will take about 15 minutes.
- Cool the breast completely. This can take anywhere from 10-30 minutes. Once cooled, cut into bite-size pieces.
- Take a large-sized bowl and stir everything except the dill and pecans together.
- Cover and chill about 1 hour before adding in dill and pecans. Serve cold.

Dinner

For dinner tonight, let's try something simple. No need for a bunch of different devices or kitchen appliances. No need for fancy spices and hours upon hours of prep. These dinner recipes are easy and accessible, yet they don't sacrifice any bit of flavor potential. They're bound to give your taste buds a delight while providing all the energy you need and fill you up for your next stint of fasting.

Single-Pan Fajita Steak

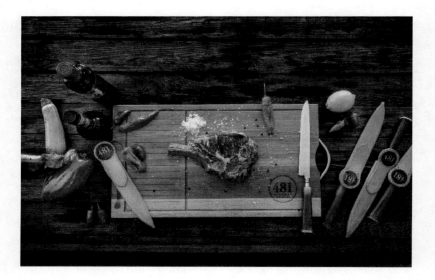

With just one sheet pan, this recipe comes together quickly and packs quite the punch for flavor! Combine it with low-carb tortillas of your choosing, eat over greens, or munch as-is. This dish is sure to please.

This recipe needs 5 minutes of prep and about 15 minutes of cooking. It will make 5 helpings.

- Fat—33 g
- Protein—31 g
- Net Carbs—5 g
- Calories—440

What to Use:

- Garlic (2 cloves, minced)
- Onion (1 medium-sized, sliced thinly)
- Chili Powder (1 teaspoon)
- Cumin (1 tablespoon)
- Salt & Pepper (to taste)
- Coconut Oil (0.25 cup)
- Lime (1, juiced & zested)
- Lemon (1, juiced & zested)
- Steak (1 pound, sliced into strips)
- Red Pepper (1 large-sized, sliced into strips)
- Yellow Pepper (1 large-sized, sliced into strips)

What to Do:

- Prepare the meat and vegetables and then stir all ingredients together on a lined or greased baking sheet.
- Preheat oven to 350 degrees then bake for 15 minutes. Half-way through the process, stir the mixture well.
- Serve with an extra sprinkle of lime juice.

Salmon Seared with Light Cream Sauce

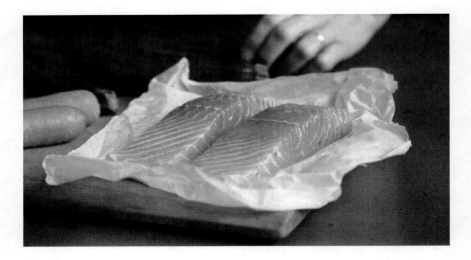

With just a handful of ingredients and a few simple steps, this recipe is gloriously easy and even more delicious than you could ever imagine. Trust me. Try it.

This recipe needs 5 minutes of prep and about 25 minutes of cooking. It will make 6 helpings.

- Fat—30 g
- Protein—54 g
- Net Carbs—2 g
- Calories—494

What to Use:

- Olive Oil (2 tablespoons)
- Salmon Fillets (3, 6-ounce fillets)
- Garlic (2 cloves, minced)
- Light Cream (1 cup)
- Cream Cheese (1 ounce)
- Capers (2 tablespoons)

- Lemon Juice (1 tablespoon)
- Dill (2 teaspoons, fresh OR 1 tablespoon, dried)
- Parmesan Cheese (2 tablespoons, grated)

What to Do:

- Grab a medium-sized skillet and heat the oil to start. Add the salmon fillets once heated through and cook 5 minutes on each side.
- Set fish aside to get the sauce together.
- In that same pan, add garlic and cook on medium heat for 2 minutes. Add cream, cream cheese, lemon juice, and capers. Simmer for 5 minutes or until thickened.
- Once thickening begins, return salmon to pan and spoon the sauce over each of the fillets.
- On low heat now, bring the salmon to the appropriate temperature. Garnish with dill and parmesan and serve!

Parmesan Bacon-Asparagus Roll-Ups

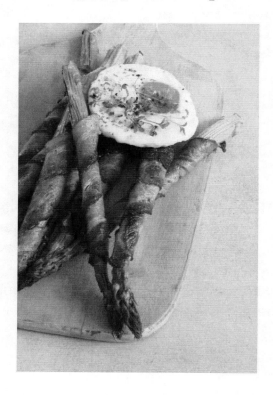

With the perfect touches of sweetness from the maple-flavored syrup and char from the baking process, these roll-ups are either the best treat ever or the perfect small meal. Enjoy as many as you like. If you need more protein than is provided in this recipe, an easy fix would be to make a chicken breast on the side. The flavor boost would be incredible with that addition, too!

This recipe needs 15 minutes of prep and about 40 minutes of cooking. It will make 2 helpings.

- Fat—23 g
- Protein—7 g
- Net Carbs—10.8 g
- Calories—257

What to Use:

- Maple-Flavored Syrup (0.5 cup)
- Butter (0.5 cup)
- Salt (0.5 teaspoon)
- Black Pepper (0.25 teaspoon)
- Asparagus (2 pounds, washed & ends removed)
- Bacon (8 slices, thick bacon)
- Parmesan (2 tablespoons + 2 teaspoons, grated)

What to Do:

- Start by preheating oven to 425 degrees.
- Then, grab a small-sized pot and bring it to medium-low heat on the stove top. Add syrup, butter, salt, and pepper. Whisk together until smooth and heated through. Set aside for later.
- Divide your 2 pounds of asparagus into 8 equal-sized groups. Wrap each group with a strip of bacon and secure the ends with toothpicks, as needed.
- Line greased baking sheet with asparagus/bacon bundles then pour over with syrup mixture and half the parmesan.
- Bake in the oven for 30 minutes. Then, switch to broil and bring the rack to the top shelf of the oven.
- Broil 2 minutes until crispy and partially-charred.
- Serve with toothpicks removed and enjoy!

Unforgettable Spaghetti Squash

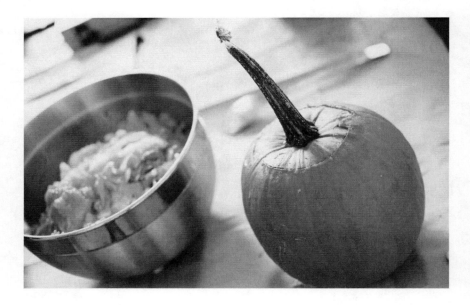

If you're like me and somewhat picky with winter squash, you're bound to be as amazed as I was when you try this spaghetti squash recipe. No pasta required, given the unique nature of this squash, and with the cheese and garlic topping, even picky eaters will surprise themselves by how much they like it. There's a little less protein in this meal than there could be, but you can boost your version by adding a little meat (try chorizo or bacon!) into the mix or by compensating through another snack or meal in the day instead.

This recipe needs 10 minutes of prep and about 1 hour of cooking. It will make 4 helpings.

- Fat—24.4 g
- Protein—8 g
- Net Carbs—3.1 g
- Calories—274

What to Use:

- Spaghetti Squash (1 medium-sized OR equivalent of 3 pounds)
- Garlic (3 cloves, minced)
- Olive Oil (1 teaspoon)
- Spinach (half-pound, chopped)
- Heavy Cream (0.5 cup)
- Parmesan Cheese (0.5 cup)
- Salt & Pepper (to taste)
- Mozzarella (grated for topping)

What to Do:

- First, preheat the oven to 400 degrees.
- Prepare the spaghetti squash by cutting it in half (lengthwise) and pulling out any seeds.
- Line a baking sheet or grease it and lay spaghetti squash with the cut side down on the sheet. Roast 30-40 minutes until easily stabbed through with a fork.
- Meanwhile, prepare the sauce. In a medium-sized pot, heat olive oil and garlic for no more than 5 minutes. Stir in spinach, cream, and parmesan in turn.
- Season with salt and pepper and set aside.
- When squash has finished roasting, pull it out from oven and begin to pull apart the strands of the squash itself (its name should make sense to you now if it didn't already!).
- With the squash threads freed, pour the cheese mixture onto the squash and into the inner "boat" part. Top with extra parmesan and mozzarella, as desired, then bake at 350 degrees for 20 additional minutes.
- At the last second, switch oven to broil and bring cheese to a beautiful browned color. Enjoy hot!

Snacks

When it comes to snacking as an Intermittent Faster, these food breaks are no joke. They're essential and important in more ways than you know. If you've chosen an IF method that relies on periodic snacks, even if you're feeling good when approaching snack time, I encourage you to *never skip those snacks*. The two listed below are packed with nutritional potential, and they're beyond easy to make. If nothing else, at least keep these two on hand, and things should be consistently productive in your IF adventure.

Hard-Boiled Eggs

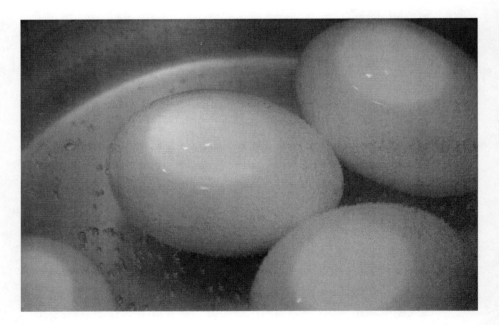

The most basic and reliable snack of all time is possibly the hard-boiled egg. With the right sprinkle of salt and pepper on top, it's hard to go wrong.

This recipe needs 5-10 minutes of cooking. It will make 4 helpings.

- Fat—29 g
- Protein—11 g
- Net Carbs—1 g
- Calories—316

What to Use:

- Eggs (8, large-sized)
- Salt & Pepper (to taste)

What to Do:

- Take a small-sized pot and fill it ¾ of the way with water. Bring to boil.
- Carefully, lay the eggs into the water and boil anywhere from 5-10 minutes. 5 minutes makes a softer egg, while 10 makes a firm and hard-boiled egg.
- Serve with topping of salt & pepper or otherwise.

Perfect Keto & IF Guacamole

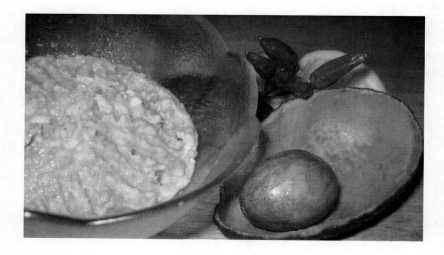

Add or subtract ingredients at will here to get your desired flavor. Going wrong with guacamole is hard! I like to add a dash of hot sauce to mine. Can't wait to see what you try. There is a little less protein than desired for proper Keto proportioning in this recipe, but you can fix that ratio with your choice of dippers or through your meal options later or earlier in the day.

This recipe needs 5-10 minutes of prep only. It will make 2 helpings.

- Fat—15 g
- Protein—3 g
- Net Carbs—13 g
- Calories—180

What to Use:

- Avocados (2 ripe ones, mashed)
- Garlic Powder (1 tablespoon)
- Onion Powder (0.5 tablespoon)

- Lime Juice (2 teaspoons)
- Salt (to taste)
- Cilantro (2 tablespoons, diced finely)
- Chili Powder or Hot Sauce (to taste)

What to Do:

- Once the avocado is mashed, stir in the garlic and onion powders along with any chili powder or hot sauce.
- As a final step, stir in lime juice and cilantro then salt to taste.
- Serve with chips or vegetable dippers!

Desserts

Dessert! The naughty word of any diet has been reclaimed in the IF / Keto Diet, for you don't always have to sacrifice treats when you're working to lose weight. The trick is to lose the carbs, stock up on fats, and add a sprinkle of protein instead. Your body will always thank you for these types of desserts, for they're designed for you to flourish (and still lose that weight!) absolutely.

No-Bake Pistachio Dessert Rounds

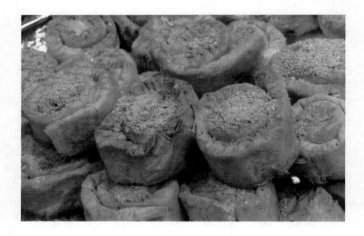

This sweet treat is easy to turn into a savory snack by just swapping out the vanilla and sweetener for garlic and fresh herbs, but it's a tasty mouth-popper either way. For dessert, this creamy and crunchy delight is sure to satisfy. As with most desserts, you lose a little by way of protein in favor of carbohydrates for this recipe, but you can make up for that with your other meals for the day, based on the method you're using.

This recipe needs 5-10 minutes of prep only. It will make 4 helpings.

- Fat—12 g
- Protein—1 g
- Net Carbs—0.5 g
- Calories—121

What to Use:

- Mascarpone Cheese (1 cup, softened)
- Vanilla Extract (0.25 teaspoon)
- Confectioner's Style Erythritol Sweetener (3 tablespoons)
- Pistachios (0.25 cup, chopped finely)

What to Do:

- In a small-sized bowl, stir together the cheese, vanilla, and sweetener. Make smooth and well-combined.
- Roll into balls. There should be about 10 1-inch diameter balls.
- Take the pistachios and chop them finely. Put onto a plate and roll the cheese balls in that pistachio powder.
- Set in refrigerator 30 minutes or more before eating. With right refrigeration, these will keep for up to one week. They will keep in the freezer for 3 months.

No-Bake Chocolate-Topped Coconut Cookies

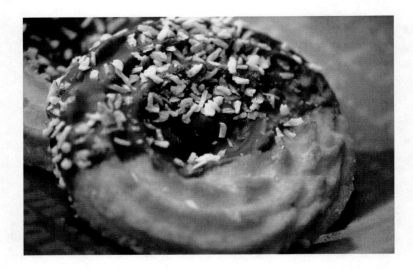

With a simple lattice of chocolate icing to top things off, these cookies are pretty to look at and even more delicious to munch on. Try and stop yourself from going back for seconds. There is a little less protein than desired for perfect Keto proportioning in this recipe, but you can balance that out by choosing a savory meal that boosts your protein and loses the carbs instead.

This recipe needs 5-10 minutes of prep. It will make 4 helpings.

- Fat—34.2 g
- Protein—3 g
- Net Carbs—8.6 g
- Calories—150

What to Use:

- Shredded Coconut (3 cups, ensure UNsweetened)
- Coconut Oil (just under 0.5 cup)
- Xylitol (0.5 cup)
- Vanilla (2 teaspoons)

- Salt (just under 0.5 teaspoon)
- Chocolate / Carob Chips (melted for drizzle)

What to Do:

- Put all ingredients except the chocolate into a blender. Process by pulsing until everything sticks together. Don't go so smooth as to make a liquid "butter" mixture.
- Once desired consistency is achieved, pour out and roll into 1-inch diameter balls. Refrigerate as desired while melting chocolate.
- Drizzle with melted chocolate in lines or a lattice. Serve chilled.

High-Protein Moussed-Up Jell-O

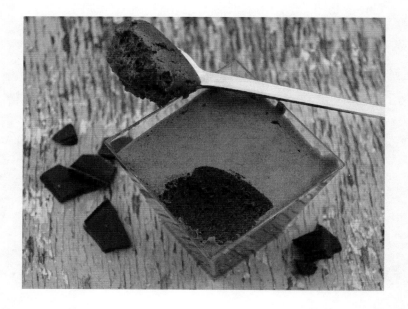

Although this recipe favors a cherry-flavored Jell-O, you can feel free to try any flavor you like! The picture above suggests chocolate, but honestly, the sky's the limit, and the outcome is just as wonderful no matter what flavor base you choose. Be sure to report back on any creative favorites!

This recipe needs 5-10 minutes of prep only. It will make 4 helpings.

- Fat—25 g
- Protein—20 g
- Net Carbs—3 g
- Calories—97

What to Use:

- Black Cherry Jell-O (1 small box, sugar-free)
- Water (0.5 cup)

- Greek Yogurt (10 ounces, plain flavored)
- Whey Protein Powder (2 scoops, unflavored)

What to Do:

- In a small-sized pot, bring water to warm yet not boiling temperature.
- Take a medium-sized mixing bowl and stir together Jell-O mix and water. Now, pour everything else into the mixing bowl and combine until perfectly smooth.
- Pour into portion bowls, ramekins, or one large bowl and refrigerate until firm, according to the Jell-O box's instructions.
- Enjoy chilled!

Conclusion

Thank you so much for making it to the end of *Intermittent Fasting*! I'm excited for you to have made it through all that information, for it means that you're ready to start putting your plans for health, diet, and growth into action. It means you should now be ready to go it on your own.

As you've been processing this information and learning all that Intermittent Fasting has to offer, you likely now have a strong and firm sense of what this dietary & lifestyle shift can do for you, and it's time to start putting all that information and all that knowledge into motion in your life.

The next step will be to make a few changes, but they don't have to be big ones! Start by just skipping the next meal! Go a day with a little less in your food portions! Begin your adjustment period into Intermittent Fasting without fear or concern, for it will be much easier and much more worthwhile than you could ever have imagined.

I am eager to hear what successes you all experience after reading this book, so please feel free to write about what happens by way of an Amazon review! You can also leave any general feedback on this book in an Amazon review, and I'd be equally appreciative. Thank you for your time and all your hard work getting ready for the Intermittent Fasting shift in your life! I can't wait to see what the future holds for you now.

Made in United States
North Haven, CT
11 September 2023

41441156R00070